Ethical Veganism, Virtue Ethics, and the Great Soul

Ethical Veganism, Virtue Ethics, and the Great Soul

Carlo Alvaro

LEXINGTON BOOKS
Lanham • Boulder • New York • London

Published by Lexington Books
An imprint of The Rowman & Littlefield Publishing Group, Inc.
4501 Forbes Boulevard, Suite 200, Lanham, Maryland 20706
www.rowman.com

6 Tinworth Street, London SE11 5AL

Copyright © 2019 by The Rowman & Littlefield Publishing Group, Inc.

All rights reserved. No part of this book may be reproduced in any form or by any electronic or mechanical means, including information storage and retrieval systems, without written permission from the publisher, except by a reviewer who may quote passages in a review.

British Library Cataloguing in Publication Information Available

Library of Congress Cataloging-in-Publication Data

Names: Alvaro, Carlo, author.
Title: Ethical veganism, virtue ethics, and the great soul / Carlo Alvaro.
Description: Lanham, MD : Lexington Books, 2019. | Includes bibliographical references and index.
Identifiers: LCCN 2019001745 (print) | LCCN 2019007072 (ebook) | ISBN 9781498590020 (Electronic) | ISBN 9781498590013 (cloth) | ISBN 9781498590037 (pbk.)
Subjects: LCSH: Animal rights. | Veganism--Moral and ethical aspects.
Classification: LCC HV4711 (ebook) | LCC HV4711 .A29 2019 (print) | DDC 179/.3--dc23
LC record available at https://lccn.loc.gov/2019001745

Contents

Preface — vii
Acknowledgments — xiii
Introduction — xv

1 Kant, Animals, and Indirect Moral Duty — 1
2 Utilitarianism: All That Is Gold Does Not Glitter — 21
3 Eating People and Eating Animals — 35
4 A New Horizon: Virtue Ethics — 51
5 What about Our Treatment of Animals? — 79
6 Veganism as a Virtue — 89
7 Some Objections — 109
8 Awareness: What We Do to Animals — 125
9 Ethical Veganism's Beef with Cultured Meat — 143

Conclusion — 165
Bibliography — 171
Index — 183
About the Author — 187

Preface

With billions of animals brought into existence and raised for food every year, the negative impact upon the environment caused by animal agriculture, the suffering experienced by those animals, cruel and redundant scientific experiments, and the staggeringly growing number of chronic diseases caused by the consumption of animal-based food, a global move toward ethical veganism is imperative. Ethical veganism is a moral position that opposes all forms of animal exploitation. This includes activities that directly hurt or kill animals, such as hunting, fishing, or animal fighting. It also includes what we support indirectly as consumers, such as eating meat and animal products, using leather, fur, and other animal by-products. Currently, it might be very hard or even impossible to avoid all products that involve some kind of animal testing or the exploitation of animals. Obviously, the goal of ethical veganism is a world in which animals are not exploited. But ethical veganism is not an all-or-nothing position; the point is to have the moral integrity to avoid as much as possible supporting animal exploitation. The proper way to understand ethical veganism is to recognize that using animals for food, research, entertainment, and more stems from lack of virtues such as compassion (feeling motivated to care for animals and not participating in practices that make animals suffer), temperance (eating for the purpose of nourishment rather than for mere taste), fairness (recognizing that it is unfair to exploit animals when it is not necessary), and magnanimity (an attitude of nobility of character that regulates all our actions, including the way we eat). My aim is to show that the acquisition of the virtues just mentioned, if correctly understood, leads to embracing ethical veganism. The virtues that I just described are concepts familiar to ethical traditions such as virtue theory, care ethics, and feminist ethics. Unlike other theories that emphasize duty, the individual, rights, and abstraction, according to these traditions morality should be done by paying attention to our moral character, relationships, care, and the particular aspects of our lives and the lives of others. The view that I propose argues that animal ethics should be framed in terms of care, compassion, and empathy toward animals; that we are already in a relationship with animals and others, and this relationship is broken and must be fixed.

Animal ethics was practically invented and further developed by moral theories that discount principles of care, compassion, empathy, and the importance of relationships. These theories, deontological and consequentialist, are still the dominant voices in the discussion of our moral obligations toward animals and nature. Unfortunately, they have devastating flaws as theories of ethics, and consequently their arguments about animals are also faulty. Worse, these theories are incapable of motivating people to do something about animal exploitation. A more promising way to construct an animal ethics, and a defense of ethical veganism, is to use the combined strengths of virtue, care, and feminist ethics because of their central values of relationship, care, empathy, compassion, temperance, attentiveness, and justice. Exercising these values in our relations with animals (and in our relations with others) involves acknowledging their moral value, thus seeing that they are not our property or food.

Our treatment of animals is morally appalling. We ought to change radically the way we live and our attitude toward animals. We must all become vegans. But what am I precisely talking about here? Considering our stage of intellectual and technological development, we could live well without having to exploit and kill other beings. And yet, hunters shoot animals for fun, farmers raise animals in cages, the meat industry slaughters animals, castrates them, debeaks them, cuts their bodies into pieces, boils them alive, drains their blood, packages their body parts, ships the packages to supermarkets where they are sold and labeled with hypocritical euphemisms such as beef, pork, drumsticks, eggs, and so on. These animal parts are bought and used as food. The reality is that people buy the mutilated body parts of cows, the cut-up flesh of pigs, the cut-off legs of chickens, and the unfertilized reproductive cycles of chickens. These animal parts are fried, broiled, roasted, and eaten—coagulated blood, skin, veins, nerves, and all, nothing gets wasted. These descriptions might sound exaggerated. But in fact the reality is even nastier. Indeed, every day the lives of millions of animals are wasted to produce meat; the process required is carefully hidden from people.

Thinking about it inevitably makes an important moral difference. Animal females—cows, for example—are forced to become pregnant. Hormones and other chemical supplements are injected into their bodies. Their babies are taken away from them and killed; their cut-up bodies are labeled and sold as veal. Chefs make a dish called "veal scaloppini," which is the name for thin slices of baby cow flesh. The cows, now engorged with milk that will never be given to their babies, since they were killed and sold as "veal," are hooked up to machines that squeeze their breasts and steal their milk. When the cows become barren and can no longer produce milk, they are sent to be slaughtered. Their milk—which, by the way, contains pus and blood—is drunk straight up or used in recipes, pus, blood, and all. The milk produced by a human mother is meant for her baby; similarly, the milk produced by a cow is meant for cow babies, not for humans, and certainly not for human adults.

For breakfast, many people eat unfertilized reproductive cycles of chickens (eggs) fried in animal lard or in the hardened artery-clogging fat of breast-squeezed animal secretion, which we call butter, with a side of fried slices of swine abdomen fat called bacon. But what really happens in egg farms? Since male chicks are not profitable because they cannot lay eggs, every year, 200 million baby chicks are ground up alive. Workers separate male chicks from females and toss the males into a chute where they are ground up alive in a meat grinder into a bloody pulp that is fed back to chickens. The industry calls this practice "instantaneous euthanasia."

For Thanksgiving dinner, millions of Americans have turkey. But are these people aware of how it is possible to have such a large number of turkeys? Turkeys naturally do not reproduce that quickly. To provide for Thanksgiving, farmers use artificial insemination. I mean that there are people whose job is to masturbate turkeys, collect the semen, and then inject it into female turkeys. (Try bringing up this as a topic next Thanksgiving dinner.)

But, as if this were not enough, animals, even insects, are used not only as food, but in countless ways in every aspect of our lives. We cover car seats with the skin of killed animals. We wash our bodies with detergents containing animal fat. We even use animal skin strips around our waists as belts and around our wrists as bracelets, or animal skin to make shoes or purses or wallets. We kill birds and use their feathers to fill up pillows and winter coats when it is absolutely unnecessary since we can use synthetic material instead. We use animal fur to make brushes and clothes, boil their bones to make Jell-O or soap, their fat to make lotions, glue, paint, or to put on our skin as lotion. Vanilla, raspberry, and strawberry ice cream flavors are enhanced by castoreum, an anal secretion of beavers! And the chewing gum you are chewing right now may contain lanolin, an oily, sweaty secretion found on the outside of sheep's wool. Lanolin is also used in skin lotions.

Insects are eaten by some cultures or utilized in many foods that people consume daily. Candies are colored using the secretions of various insects or using crushed bugs. Another insect product that many people consume daily without giving it any thought is insect vomit. Commercially, the acidic vomit of bees is known as "honey." Honey is bees' food. Obviously, the stolen honey, which is food for the hive, must be replaced. Bees must then rely on high fructose corn syrup, which is not the bee's natural food. The reliance of bees on corn syrup may be the cause of the death of millions of colonies worldwide. Just think about it. There are animal parts and animal by-products everywhere—in toothpaste, in breakfast, in pockets, around people's necks, in cars—animals, animals, and more animals. In other words, not a day goes by without humans using the dead bodies of animals and insects. In animal ethics, typically the discussion revolves around the utility of animals or their status or their rights. But we seldom pause to reflect on our moral character: What kind of individuals are those who support such disgraceful practices? Have they not compassion to realize that using animals is callous? Have they not temperance to resist consuming animal-based food, which is not essential for human health?

But animals are not only killed, eaten, or used, but also tortured while alive. Every minute, every day, hundreds of animals are killed in laboratories in the United States. Millions are used in experiments and die every year. Many animals die after being administered drugs or cosmetics. The government requires testing on animals before products are sold to people. But consider that many natural cosmetic products on the market are not required to be tested on animals. Ask yourself, why do we need to test toothpaste or mascara on animals when we can produce and use only natural cosmetics that do not require animal testing at all? And since humans "need" these products, why don't they test them on humans? There is more: In a recent experiment, baboons were strapped down and had special helmets cemented to their skulls. Then, a pneumatic device delivered calibrated blows to determine the strength of the helmet. The blows continued until the skull of the baboons were fractured, resulting in the death of the baboons. Dogs are driven to the point of insanity by electric shocks so that scientists can study the effect of insanity. Cats are deprived of sleep until they die to study sleep deprivation. Elephants were given LSD to study its effects. Mice had their legs cut off to study how they walk on their stumps. Polar bears were drowned in vats filled with oil to study the effects of oil spills in polar regions. Cats were blinded, castrated, and rendered deaf to study their sexual developments under these incapacities. Other cats are placed in small rooms heated up to 110 degrees Fahrenheit and left there until they die. This process produces a musk in the cats' genitals, which is scraped off and used in the production of perfume, making the scent last longer.

Meat eaters say that they enjoy meat. But just because one enjoys something does not make what one does moral. You may "enjoy" your steak or chicken dish, but have you ever considered that your few minutes of enjoyment gave those animals a miserable life ended by a brutal death?

It might be believed that eating meat is not immoral because it is the cycle of life. Perhaps that's true. But the reality, however, is that people buy meat in supermarkets because it would be very time and energy consuming to try to hunt our food. Animals have to be transformed into food. This transformation involves separation, fear, death, blood, and bad odor; it involves cutting up the flesh, packaging, seasoning, and cooking. At the end of this process, the final product is no longer an animal. This very process creates a distance, or an absence. As Carol J. Adams puts it, "Behind every meal of meat is an absence: the death of the animal whose place the meat takes. This is the 'absent referent.'"[1] Our interactions with these creatures do not make one hungry because animals are not our food—fruits and plants are our food. Animals are creatures with desires, friends, families, and the desire to thrive and not to be imprisoned and killed to become food or shoes or purses. They are, most importantly, creatures with which we have a bond. Many people have companion animals that they love. Unfortunately, the love for these creatures is not consistent; some animals are considered friends while others are food.[2]

But since animals eat other animals, why would it be wrong for us to eat animals as well? Carnivores like lions, tigers, and hyenas do not have a choice; nature "designed" them to eat the flesh of other animals. They cannot survive solely on plant food—we can. In fact, we do better with plant food. Also, it does not seem to be a fair analogy because humans and carnivores obtain their food in quite different ways. Carnivores do not walk into supermarkets, buy steaks, season them, and grill them. They catch their food and eat the whole animal, flesh, hair, eyes, blood, bones, and nerves, right there on the spot—people buy meat in supermarkets.

Eating animals is not essential for good health. In fact, science is very clear about the danger of consuming animal products—that is, they are unhealthful. Research has decisively shown that eating meat and dairy products causes heart disease, diabetes, obesity, atherosclerosis formation, cancer, and more, and that a plant-based diet not only lowers, but also in many cases reverses, those conditions.[3]

Our treatment of animals should make us reflect upon the purpose of our life on this planet. The way history has unfolded makes us care about only our immediate surroundings. In so doing, humans have killed not only other humans but also animals, and we are destroying the environment. Thus, I believe that changing our attitude toward animals—that is, acknowledging that they are not our property and our food—is a way to reconnect with nature and the rest of the world. It is also a way to remind us that we are guests on earth, and not hosts. And since we pride ourselves in having the capacity of reason, which allows us to create, among other things, sophisticated ethical systems, we should accept this fact and use that capacity to realize that exploiting animals is unnecessary and therefore wrong.

In the foregoing, I have described only some of the absurdities and the evil that humans unnecessarily inflict upon animals. There are many other horrific examples. My hope is that these examples suffice to strike a chord with people and make them realize that human exploitation of animals is no more justified than the exploitation of other people. My hope is that people realize the moral necessity to end what I call the world's greatest injustice toward nature: exploiting animals. The only morally consistent way to live is to become ethical vegans, which, in practical terms, means to stop eating animal flesh, cease using animal by-products, and shun all products obtained through animal testing. The way to move in that direction, in my view, is to change the way we do morality. Namely, we should abandon deontic and consequentialist principles and embrace instead virtue-based values.

NOTES

1. Carol J. Adams, *The Sexual Politics of Meat: A Feminist-Vegetarian Critical Theory* (New York: Bloomsbury Academic, 2015).

2. This point is made by Melanie Joy in *Why We Love Dogs, Eat Pigs, and Wear Cows: An Introduction to Carnism* (Boston: Conari Press, 2011).

3. W. J. Craig and A. R. Mangels, "Position of the American Dietetic Association: Vegetarian Diets," *Am. Diet Assoc.* 109, no. 7 (July 2009): 1266–82. Also, in 2015, twenty-two scientists from the World Health Organization (WHO)'s International Agency for Research on Cancer (IARC) evaluated over eight hundred medical studies and concluded that consumption of processed meat is "carcinogenic to humans," and that consumption of red meat is "probably carcinogenic to humans." Their conclusions were based on overwhelming evidence for positive associations between meat and colorectal cancer, as well as positive associations between processed meat consumption and stomach cancer, and between red meat consumption and pancreatic and prostate cancer. See http://www.iarc.fr/en/media-centre/pr/2015/pdfs/pr240_E.pdf.

Acknowledgments

First I would like to thank my wife Malaika for her constant encouragement and loving support through all the years that we have been together. And I thank my children George, Jon, and Valentina for giving me unconditional love. Also, I would like to thank many people who have helped me write this book in various ways, including my past teachers and students. I thank Igor Sotgiu; Daniel Capruso; Gregory Tague; Laura Mucci (Grazie per aver sempre creduto in me); Paul Kelly; Ira Greene; Alan Redner; Rocco, Teresa, and Alessandro Alvaro; Carullo Carmela; Maria and Mauro Polese; Joshua Barash; Roberto Ripollino; Zed Adams; Alice Crary; Dimitri Nikulin; John Noras; Zenon Feszczak; Tyler Perkins; and Joanne Zeller.

Introduction

The aim of this book is to provide moral grounds for what I call ethical veganism. The term "veganism" is often associated with diet, perhaps due to the sudden interest in veganism and its popularity among Hollywood stars. However, ethical veganism is the moral view according to which, in most cases where access to plant-based alternatives is readily available, we ought to avoid using animals as a source of food, clothing, and by-products, such as eggs, dairy, honey, leather, fur, silk, wool, cosmetics, animal-derived detergents, and more. I argue that, in general, eating animals is a disgraceful practice. I can sense the immediate reaction of the reader upon reading my last statement. One may point out that there are many circumstances in which eating or killing an animal is not disgraceful. This is partly true. But as I will discuss later, such circumstances are typically illustrations of extreme states of affairs. For example, in 2016, the Cincinnati Zoo shot and killed a four-hundred-pound gorilla named Harambe after a four-year-old child fell into the gorilla's enclosure. Harambe dragged the child around for roughly ten minutes. Assuming that Harambe would eventually kill the child, zoo officials decided to kill the animal. Did the zoo official not do the right thing? It would seem to be the case. Another classic example is eating animals if stranded on a desert island or populations who live in places where plant-based food is not available. I will address this issue in the course of my discussion, but for now I wish to make one remark: Extreme circumstances certainly can force individuals to act in ways that, under normal circumstances, would be considered immoral. Certainly most would agree that the zoo officials would have done something immoral had they shot Harambe to retrieve, say, a wallet that had fallen into the animal's quarter. Conversely, most people would say that when the four-year-old child fell into the animal's enclosure, and the gorilla threatened the child's life, shooting the animal was the right thing to do. To put it differently, most would say that the zoo official did not do anything that could be considered immoral. However, it does not follow that his action was admirable. This rationale might strike the reader as confusing. I think the problem stems from the fact that our moral language is, after all, a product of a moral attitude that I reject. What I reject is a morality according to which once we understand our duty, we also can determine that an action in accordance to our duty is right and not performing it is wrong.[1] In my view, this general description of what counts as a right action is incomplete. It seems to me that there are many actions that are objectively wrong, and that no circumstance could make them right. One might argue that the action in question is the only one available or the best possible one, but again, being necessary or being the only available option does not make an action right. In other words, the end may be said to justify the means, but it cannot be said that the end transforms a wrong action into a right one. As Rosalind Hursthouse notes, a person can make the right decision given the circumstances, but by no means is that decision the right thing to do.[2] For these reasons, I prefer to use terms such as "virtuous" or "admirable" or "despicable" or "disgraceful" to describe an action, rather than using "moral" or "immoral." In the case of the morality of using animals for food and other purposes, I want to argue that a circumstance may require that an animal be killed or eaten, but the act of killing or eating does not switch its nature from bad to good or from disgraceful to admirable or from wrong to right.

The view I present is not the starting point of my argument, but rather the conclusions of my general view on morality. My view on morality in general is very similar to that proposed by Aristotle (384–322 BCE)—the view that a moral person is one who acts virtuously. Like Aristotle, I believe that the ultimate goal of humans is to be happy, and happiness is achieved through a life of virtue. What I mean by this statement is something that I will need to articulate more precisely later. The idea, however, is to have an accomplished life, a life with which one could be satisfied. One important aspect of each individual life is the actions that one performs. Actions may differ from one individual to another, but the final goal of achieving an accomplished life is the same for everyone. What I will argue here is that to accomplish such a life, an individual must act virtuously. For the moment, it is sufficient to say that what I mean by "acting virtuously" is simply what most people regard as being just, compassionate, temperate, magnanimous, and more. Later, I will try to explain what exactly it is to be just, compassionate, temperate, magnanimous, and so on, and why it is necessary or even desirable to have these moral characteristics. To be more specific, a life of deception, greed, callousness, unfriendliness, and so on could be to some extent beneficial to an individual. But by no means does it follow that it will lead to a flourishing life. And since I believe that our eating habits are actions that matter morally,

I argue that our eating habits ought to be virtuous actions, and consequently they should be the expression of justice, compassion, temperance, and magnanimity. As it will emerge from my discussion, ethical veganism is thus an expression of virtue. Such a view acknowledges that we are not perfect but that we have a responsibility to try our best to avoid using animals.

My moral outlook offers an alternative approach to the Singer/Regan argument against animal exploitation. I propose a virtue-oriented approach. By saying "the Singer/Regan argument," I refer to the two well-known ethical theories of consequentialism and deontology, which have been the dominating forces behind the animal rights movement. My aim is to show that (a) embracing these theories is counterproductive to the accomplishment of the goals they try to achieve; and (b) if those goals—namely liberating animals—are desired, it is necessary to perform a paradigm shift from the current view of morality to a virtue-oriented approach. The shift I have in mind here is a shift in the way we look at the question of our relationship with and obligation toward animals. Such a paradigm shift can make us realize the importance of what I call ethical veganism—that is, the moral position according to which, in most cases, if not all, using animals for food and other purposes is unvirtuous. Unlike many previous arguments in favor of veganism/vegetarianism, I do not wish to argue that it is immoral to use animals because they have rights, or because animals can contribute to the aggregate pleasure/happiness. It seems that many moral philosophers are interested only in what our actions can achieve or whether our actions follow certain rules. But in so doing they overlook or discount the importance of individual moral character. It seems that such theories are more interested in people acting justly, honestly, and compassionately than in people being just, honest, and compassionate.

In fact, my motivation for writing this is that virtue ethics has a wealth of insights that can motivate people to become vegans. Why is this important? In recent years, it has become overwhelmingly evident that veganism offers many benefits: It can prevent or reverse certain health conditions, such as heart disease and type 2 diabetes.[3] It avoids wasting resources. At present, we could have enough food to feed ten billion people, more people than the ones in this world. Animals raised for food—which are brought into existence by humans—are eating 50 percent of grains worldwide, while 82 percent of children are starving. As an example of the waste of food, approximately 70 percent of the grain grown in the United States alone is fed to livestock; this amount of grain is enough to feed 800 million people.[4] There is also the problem of water wasted to produce animal products. It has been estimated that being vegans could save up to 724,925 gallons of water per person each year.[5] Regarding human health, the hormones found in animal products can cause cancer development,[6] and "high meat availability is correlated to increased prevalence of obesity."[7] Eating meat and animal products is unnecessary. While the animals' rights movement and other likeminded commentators have been churning out books and articles arguing that using animals is immoral, the spectacular fact is that no serious argument has ever been produced in support of using animals for food. Animals are raised, killed, and eaten simply for pleasure or tradition. Typically, using animals has been morally justified by arguing about the nutritional value of animal-based products. However, the notion that animal-based food is healthful or essential is demonstrably false. Consumption of meat and animal products is unnecessary. There is no evidence that human beings must eat meat, dairy, or eggs in order to be healthy. In fact, the opposite is the case.[8] Furthermore there is evidence that raising animals for food is not sustainable and is the cause of environmental degradation.[9]

While it is true that both consequentialists and deontologists take the scientific findings just mentioned to heart, such theories can merely point their fingers at these facts and suggest their respective preferred moral approaches: We all believe (I hope) that it is wrong for human beings to pollute and destroy the natural environment and to waste natural resources—but wrong it what sense? Is it because a sustainable environment is essential to human well-being? Or is it wrong because nature has intrinsic value that ought to be respected? John Nolt notes that many arguments that try to show us we have certain obligations toward nature rely on a conception that nature is a good.

> Each good that we find in nature is a good *for* some natural entities. Adequate sunlight is a good *for* photosynthetic plants; preference-satisfaction may be good *for* a sentient being that has desires; reproductive success is (up to a certain point) good *for* a species. . . . But why should the goods of those entities obligate us?[10]

Raising animals for food has caused, and continues to cause, ecological disasters. What we need to avert this, I argue, is the adoption of a different moral outlook. Neither utilitarianism nor deontology can account for the wrongness of wantonly destroying our environment. What I propose is that change in our attitudes toward nature will come from a different approach to morality. It is more profitable, then, to address these practices by recognizing what is wrong with our moral character. The practices described above stem from the vices of greed—self-indulgence expressed by a defective moral character. The satisfaction of aggregate preference, duty, and rights, no doubt, are important moral aspects, but without the acquisition of virtuous character, it is like putting the proverbial cart before the horse: We are not likely to produce the results that other theories try to achieve by starting from the questions of what actions will maximize utility or what is my duty and the right action.

One aspect of virtue ethics in particular that enables us to see what is vicious about some of our attitudes toward nature is what Aristotle calls the crown of the virtues—that is, greatness of soul—which he discusses in *Nicomachean Ethics*, Book IV.3. A great-souled individual possesses great moral qualities, such as compassion, temperance, and a sense of what is right or wrong in a given circumstance. A great-souled individual is "the sort of person to do good," and "it would be quite unfitting [for such an individual] to run away with his arms swinging, or to commit an injustice."[11] The kind of picture we get of the great-souled individual is a magnanimous and just individual who cares about others and who "tends to produce or to preserve happiness."[12] Being just means avoiding actions in accordance with vice, such as wanton violence.[13] It would seems plausible, then, that given the potential harm to the environment caused by intensive animal farming, a great-souled person will, for example, avoid the products of intensive animal farming.

Furthermore, my aim is to articulate veganism; and by explaining certain features of virtue ethics, I want to show what is admirable and worth embracing about veganism. Typically, veganism is promoted by organizations such as PETA, the Vegan Society, and other animal rights organizations, but it is never properly defended. For example, according to thoughtco.com, "Veganism is the practice of minimizing harm to all animals, which requires abstention from animal products, such as meat, fish, dairy, eggs, honey, gelatin, lanolin, wool, fur, silk, suede and leather."[14] The language used is "minimize" and "requires abstention." But one should not become a vegan only because it minimizes harm, and certainly not simply because it is a requirement or abstention. This attitude suggests that one might enjoy eating meat and other animal products but forces himself not to do it. This is the wrong attitude. One should not be motivated to be a vegan by such principles; rather, one should be internally motivated by a virtuous character and by observing the lives of animals and their objective moral characteristics. Not surprisingly, the very People for the Ethical Treatment of Animals (PETA) say, "we would not oppose eating eggs from chickens treated as companions if the birds receive excellent care and are not purchased from hatcheries."[15]

I want to propose that veganism is an expression of moral virtue. Virtues are not innate, but are acquired through practice. They are states of character that find expression in actions conducive to a good life. A virtuous individual avoids both excess and defect. A temperate person, for example, will avoid eating too much or too little, but will also avoid eating things that are not food, that are not necessary, and that are deleterious for her health. Now take eggs, for example. Hens ovulate to reproduce, just like humans. Chicken eggs that are sold as food are the result of hens' unfertilized reproductive cycles. They are used as food—but they are actually unfertilized reproductive cycles. Consider also that chickens are the result of centuries of domestication and genetic manipulation. They spend their lives in farms where life for them is not as good as it can be. Considering that chickens are very sensitive animals and this process in most cases prevents them from flourishing, not unreasonably, it follows that a compassionate individual does not eat eggs, nor is he interested in eating them—even those laid from "happy" chickens.

John Stuart Mill said that every great movement is first ridiculed, then discussed, and eventually adopted. The idea that animals enter the world of morality was ridiculed to the point that thinkers of the caliber of Descartes argued that animals are mere automata.[16] Then came the animal rights movement led by Peter Singer and Tom Regan, with many others following in their footsteps. They made the world discuss veganism. But the third stage, adoption, is being delayed. Millions of animals are still artificially inseminated and give birth to animals that people exploit. These animals are very peaceful and sensitive beings. Sadly, they are caged, separated from their parents and children, debeaked, castrated, killed, skinned, suffocated, anally electrocuted, turned into food, paint, glue, shoes, soap, and shaving brushes, and they are used as subjects of horrific and painful scientific research. As if this were not enough, bringing into existence so many animals and raising them exacerbates already serious environmental problems, such as global warming caused by the emission of greenhouse gases. These animals also produce an enormous amount of waste that pollutes our waterways and contributes to deforestation and wastewater. They also consume valuable plant food that could feed many people who lack proper nutrition.

Furthermore, when we look at what health sciences have to say about eating meat, we find overwhelming evidence that a meat-based diet causes a number of chronic diseases, while a vegan approach avoids, prevents, and in many cases even reverses such conditions. This is a serious ethical problem: humans eat animals, hunt them, experiment on them, wear their furs and skins, and more. All these practices are done before our eyes and noses without our realizing their viciousness. These practices are self-destructive, cruel, and immoral without our realizing it. The solution to these problems is for us to become vegans—that is, for people to stop regarding animals as property or food. Veganism is the only morally consistent position with respect to our relationship with other animals and the environment. By veganism, I understand a virtuous attitude toward animals that sees animals as creatures that exist for their own benefit and are not humans' property or sources of food.

Our treatment of animals, and its resulting effects upon the environment, is vicious, unjust, and also self-destructive. So why the delay? The answer is very complex, but the beginning of an answer is that the wrong advocates for animals have been discussing the question of how we treat non-human animals. To be fair, we must acknowledge that philosophers such as Peter Singer and Tom Regan have to be given credit for bringing to light the discussion and urging us to question the morality of our relationship with animals. However, their essentialist approach has serious limitations that caused the delay of acceptance. Their arguments, which rely upon utilitarian calculations of overall preferences (Singer), rights (Regan), or duty (Korsgaard), are incapable of motivating us to accept the abolition of factory farming, hunting, and animal experimentation. These accounts only go so far as granting vegetarianism.

Regan and others rely on conceptions of rights and duty that are flawed. Regan argues that we should focus on the similarities and not the differences between animals and us. Both Regan and Singer, though they propose different ethical accounts, share the idea that there is no morally relevant difference between animals and humans that could justify animal exploitation. So Regan argues that because animals are subject of a life like humans in the sense that they feel and have desires and a variety of experiences just like us, and because they can be harmed just like humans, they also have a value that should be respected. The difficulty with these types of arguments is that the symmetry they propose between human and non-human animals is questionable. Perhaps it is a form of anthropomorphism to argue that our experiences are similar to those of animals in a way that is irrelevant to morality. As a matter of fact, many people find this symmetry argument unconvincing and are unmoved toward veganism. The trouble is that while it is true that animals suffer, this is not, by itself, enough to show that humans and animals are relevantly similar so that human and animal suffering should have equal moral importance.[17]

I offer a more promising approach that relies on the combined forces of virtue ethics, care ethics, and feminist ethics, all of which I consider expressions of virtue. These ethics focus on the differences rather than the similarities between animals and humans. This is important for at least two reasons: the first is that considering the differences between humans and animals opens our understanding to the uniqueness and value of each individual, which is typically obscured by the generalization of traditional or non-aretaic ethics. And the second is that the acknowledgement of these differences encourages us to pay close attention to others and develop an internal motivation to respond to the needs of others; this in turn enables us to acquire a virtuous character. As it will emerge from my discussion, morality is about having a noble character. What we do to animals, any way we word it or try to justify, is ignoble. Consequently, my thesis here is that all humans should stop regarding animals as property and become vegans, that is, stop buying, and eating animal flesh, dairy products, using animal by-products, and products obtained through animal testing.

Traditional ethical approaches, such as utilitarianism, deontology, and rights theory, fail to move us in the right direction because they focus on abstract, detached, or legalistic concepts; moreover, they suggest that we do not rely upon our natural emotions such as empathy and compassion. But if we do not acquire a virtuous character and follow abstract principles instead, then we will never see the wrongness of regarding animals as property, will never be motivated to become vegans. The advantage of an ethics of virtue is that an individual does what is just, compassionate, temperate, and generous because her character internally motivates her. Properly understood, virtue ethics entails veganism.

To show why ethical veganism is the natural expression of a virtuous character, I first show that non-aretaic theories, such as deontology and consequentialism, with their focus on extending equal consideration of rights, in fact undermine the goals they try to achieve. I then propose a virtue-based approach and claim that it is superior to other approaches. Virtue ethics, the feminist tradition, and care ethics form a cumulative argument showing that moral growth is impossible unless we focus on character and relationship with others. To the objection that virtue and care ethics can only go so far as making us concerned about a restricted circle of beings, I show that this is not true. In fact, when we acquire and apply in particular the virtues of compassion, fairness, temperance, and greatness of soul, we will be motivated to care about non-human animals that are outside our circle of care. Social forces deliberately hinder our capacity to acquire these virtues and motivate ourselves to care for others by obscuring our true perception of what is done to animals. Virtue and care are capable of moving us to become ethical vegans by making us acknowledge particular important facts about ourselves and the lives of animals and what is done to them by science, farming, and hunting, but also by those who have a latent prejudice that makes them regard animals as things that can be milked, used, or regulated.

I begin my discussion by considering Kant's position with regard to our treatment of animals—not a very reassuring one, to be sure. This position is known as the "indirect duty view." It says that we have no direct duties toward animals simply because they lack reason and are incapable of imposing moral laws on us. I also consider Tom Regan and Christine Korsgaard's neo-Kantian accounts on the question of our treatment of animals. I engage with these positions and conclude that both Kant's view and neo-Kantian views are flawed and thus not able to address the immorality of our treatment of animals.

I next consider utilitarianism and show that it cannot deliver what it promises. As I mentioned previously, utilitarian theories are internally inconsistent because on the one hand they urge us to consider that we are doing something wrong to animals, but on the other hand, by its very definition, utilitarianism is open to exploiting animals or people so long as it maximizes utility. Worse, according to utilitarianism, the lives of animals or humans are not special in any way, except for the fact that they have preferences that can be satisfied or frustrated. So, as it turns out, utilitarianism is concerned about animals, but only insofar as their preferences are satisfied and contribute to overall happiness; or, in other words, utilitarianism is not concerned about animals themselves as valuable individual beings having moral characteristics.

Having shown that the prevailing theories, which are very vocal about the wrongness of our treatment of non-human animals, fail to deliver what they promise, I try to spell out more precisely what is problematic with such theories as a way to discuss the superiority of an ethic of virtue. Here I discuss virtue ethics and its components and how cultivating certain virtues, especially compassion, temperance, and fairness, enables us to see what is virtuous about veganism. I take this ethical approach especially in arguing for a normative virtue ethics and the idea of care as a virtue. I conclude by asking whether we can use virtue ethics/ethics of care to criticize meat eating. Having considered a range of views, I argue that the right answer is yes.

Later, I present my main argument for why we should all become vegans. My argument is an application of virtue/care ethics. Here I claim that if we acquire in particular the virtues of temperance, compassion, fairness (which is an expression of the virtues of justice), and greatness of soul, we inevitably find that the only morally consistent attitude toward animals is to be ethical vegans. I discuss the application of virtue ethics with regard to our relationships with animals and with regard to the environment. I argue that not just vegetarianism but ethical veganism is an expression of virtuous character. The transition from virtue to veganism is almost automatic as we consider the differences between humans and animals I mentioned earlier. In my view, vegetarianism is not an option because it still involves practices that are just vicious or lack virtue because they involve cruelty, indifference, disrespect of animals, and unfairness. Also, I consider the prospect of raising animals "humanely" or cruelty free. I argue that this is playing with words and really offensive to the moral integrity of a virtuous character; moreover, it is offensive to the animals that in the end are killed and have their bodily parts and secretions used for food and more. The only solution to fix our relationship with animals is for us to be or become ethical vegans. For most people in the world, eating animal products, such as meat, dairy, and more, is not necessary, and therefore it goes against what is compassionate, fair, temperate, and against the integrity of a magnanimous character. Furthermore, thanks to the abundance and prosperity of many countries in the world, nowadays it is possible to feed and clothe the whole planet, including the less fortunate, without using any animal products.

Successively, I survey the nutritional landscape in arguing that health sciences do not speak for eating meat. In fact, I present some of the most recent scientific studies, all of which undisputedly show that consuming animal products causes such chronic diseases and conditions as atherosclerosis, obesity, heart disease, diabetes, and more. On the contrary, there is good evidence that a plant-based diet is more healthful. In other words, eating animals is wrong, among other reasons, because it is a useless, self-destructive, and self-indulging practice. I conclude with the considerations that eating and using animals causes a great deal of preventable pollution and damage to the environment, and it wastes food and water that could be given to people who are starving and have no access to clean water.

Additionally, as an important aspect of my argument, I claim that we have a distorted view of animals, inculcated in us in deliberately manipulative ways, which prevents us from regarding animals as creatures that deserve moral respect and from acquiring virtue. I argue that our current relationship with animals, which sees them as property, is immoral. What is peculiar about our relationship with animals is that we are capable of respecting animals, but at the same time we regard them as food and property. On this score, I consider the root of this moral discrepancy and possible ways of reaching people to inform them in a non-manipulative way. The main issue is that there are strong political and social interests perpetrating animal exploitation. The meat industry achieves this by using deliberately manipulative language that permeates our culture through the media. As I point out, education should take into consideration how animal exploitation is hidden, downplayed, or glorified. I also suggest the use of art and literature as a way to bring to light important moral characteristics that animals possess, which are otherwise obscured by euphemisms and simplifications.

NOTES

1. Here I am referring to deontology, according to which doing my duty means that if I act according to duty my action is right even if someone else thinks it is not. The classical example is that of Kant saying that one should not lie even to protect others' lives. I am not elaborating this example here because I will do so in my discussion of Kantian ethics in chapter 1. Utilitarianism, though different from deontology in many respects, also argues that an action is right if it can lead to the greatest good for the greatest number. Thus, if I perform that action I am guaranteed that action is right, and in no sense is the action wrong.
2. See Hursthouse, *On Virtue Ethics* (Oxford: Oxford University Press, 1999), 78. Also, for a further discussion of the distinction between right and moral, see Liezel Van Zyl, "Virtue Ethics and Right Action," in *The Cambridge Companion to Virtue Ethics* (Cambridge: Cambridge University Press, 2013).
3. See https://www.health.harvard.edu/heart-health/halt-heart-disease-with-a-plant-based-oil-free-diet-. Also see https://www.ncbi.nlm.nih.gov/pubmed/19562864.
4. UNICEF, "Improving Child Nutrition," https://www.unicef.org/gambia/Improving_Child_Nutrition_the_achievable_imperative_for_global_progress.pdf.
5. See https://www.ewg.org/meateatersguide/interactive-graphic/water/.
6. See http://www.pcrm.org/health/cancer-resources/diet-cancer/facts/meat-consumption-and-cancer-risk.
7. W. You and M. Henneberg, "Meat Consumption Providing a Surplus Energy in Modern Diet Contributes to Obesity Prevalence," *BMC Nutr.* 2 (2016): 22. https://doi.org/10.1186/s40795-016-0063-9.

8. "Nutritional Update for Physicians: Plant-Based Diets," https://www.ncbi.nlm.nih.gov/pmc/articles/PMC3662288/.

9. See the following articles: http://www.worldwatch.org/files/pdf/Livestock%20and%20Climate%20Changepdf; https://academic.oup.com/ajcn/article/78/3/660S/4690010; http://www.earthsave.org/environment/foodchoices.htm; http://science.sciencemag.org/content/314/5800/787.

10. John Nolt, "The Move from Good to Ought," *Environmental Ethics* 28, no. 4 (Winter 2006): 355–374. DOI: 10.5840/enviroethics20062843.

11. Aristotle, *Nichomachean Ethics* (Cambridge: Cambridge University Press, 2000), IV.3, 1123b, 30, 1124b, 18.

12. Ibid., 1129b, 18.

13. Ibid., V. 1129b, 21.

14. ThoughtCo., "What Is Veganism?"

15. "Is It OK to Eat Eggs from Chickens I've Raised in My Backyard?" http://www.peta.org/about-peta/faq/is-it-ok-to-eat-eggs-from-chickens-ive-raised-in-my-backyard/.

16. In a letter to the Marquess of Newcastle, Descartes explains that non-language-having animals cannot be rational beings. He writes, "I cannot share the opinion of Montaigne and others who attribute understanding or thought to animals," for none of our external actions can show "that our body is not just a self-moving machine but contains a soul with thoughts, with the exception of words, or other signs." For Descartes, humans and animals differ in kind rather than in degree. Animals are mere automata, and their behavior can be explained in terms of the laws of physics, and not thought.

17. A similar objection is made by Brian Luke in "Justice, Caring and Animal Liberation," in *The Feminist Care Tradition in Animal Ethics*, ed. Josephine Donovan and Carol J. Adams (New York: Columbia University Press, 2007), 124–148.

Chapter One

Kant, Animals, and Indirect Moral Duty

Kant thought that human beings are morally special. He thought that humans possess an intrinsic moral worth that makes them the most important beings in creation. All other animals, according to Kant, do not have intrinsic value; they are not morally important in themselves, but rather have instrumental value as they serve human purpose. One way to describe Kant's moral view is that rational beings are ends in themselves, while non-rational ones are only means to the ends of rational beings. Humans are special because they have desires and goals. When we think about certain animals, we often remark how beautiful and intelligent they are, how affectionate they are, and how many other humanlike characteristics they possess. For example, chimpanzees seem to have a moral understanding of the suffering of others. They have been observed saving other chimpanzees from drowning. And in an experiment where rhesus monkeys had to choose between getting food by pulling a chain that would deliver an electric shock to a companion or not getting food and starving themselves for several days, they chose to starve and avoid causing harm to their companions.[1]

It seems unlikely that Kant knew about these experiments. But I suspect that even if he had known about them, he would not have been impressed by them as much as many are nowadays. Kant was interested in the question of moral obligation and of duty. Some animals seem to exhibit moral behavior, but that is not enough to consider them moral beings. I am not suggesting that Kant was a behaviorist. It is not the behavior of beings that is important in Kant's moral view, but rather rationality. Kant argued that non-human animals are not rational in the sense that they lack the capacity to legislate and enforce moral laws. To be rational for Kant, a being must be capable of giving himself rules and acting upon them; he must have free will. People can freely make decisions and set goals in their lives; animals cannot. Consequently, they are the locus of moral value. If people did not exist, morality would not exist.

Descartes (1596–1650) argues that because animals lack reason, they do not feel pain; Descartes regarded animals as organic automata. For Descartes, only humans feel pain. They have minds and souls, and therefore only humans deserve compassion. For Kant, non-human animals (henceforth referred to as animals) are not just mere automata as Descartes argued. Kant recognized that animals feel pain, but thought that they are not rational and they lack free will; they obey the laws of nature like other things in nature. They are, most importantly, not capable of giving themselves rules upon which they can act. They cannot legislate their behavior or impose laws upon others. Thus, they are not *direct* members of the moral community. Therefore, rational beings, such as rational, competent humans, have no direct moral duty toward animals. Nevertheless, Kant argued that we should try to be kind to animals—but for our own sake, not theirs. He argued that being cruel to animals makes humans become cruel to each other; conversely, being good to them fosters good behavior toward other human beings.

> If a man shoots his dog because the animal is no longer capable of service, he does not fail in his duty to the dog, for the dog cannot judge, but his act is inhuman and damages in himself that humanity which it is his duty to show towards mankind. If he is not to stifle his human feelings, he must practice kindness towards animals, for he who is cruel to animals becomes hard also in his dealings with men.[2]

Kant claimed that we do not have any direct duties toward animals. In Kant's *Lectures on Ethics*, he clearly states that since animals are not rational beings, we have no moral duties to them: "[So] far as animals are concerned, we have no direct duties. Animals are not self-conscious and are there merely as the means to an end. That end is man. . . . Our duties towards animals are merely indirect duties towards humanity."[3] Again, in this passage Kant emphasizes that rationality is the ground of morality and the basis of personhood; but since, according to Kant, animals are not rational, they are not persons, and consequently we do not have any moral duties toward them.

> The fact that the human being can have the representation "I" raises him infinitely above all the other beings on earth. By this he is a person . . . that is, a being altogether different in rank and dignity from things, such as irrational animals, with which one may deal and dispose at one's discretion.[4]

A straightforward reading of these and other such passages may suggest that Kant had no regard for animals' welfare at all. In other words, when it comes to animal advocacy, Kantian ethics is not regarded as a favorable ethical system to vindicate the rights of animals. However, several Kantian scholars have offered careful examinations of Kant's moral theory to show that this is not the case. They point out that Kantian ethics has a lot to say about our treatment of animals, and that Kant's theory, by showing that we have indirect duties toward them, makes a strong case for treating animals with respect.

As the above quotations indicate, Kant was very clear about duties: We have *direct* duties *only* toward rational beings. Having *direct* duties toward a being means that we have a moral obligation toward him. What does this mean? For Kant it means that since human beings are intrinsically valuable, we have a moral obligation to treat them with respect. We must treat other people well, avoid harming them and lying to them, and respect their rights. We must treat people as ends rather than as means to our ends. This implies that we should not use or exploit a person for our own benefit. For example, let's say that I am in desperate need of money and ask you to lend me some; I promise that I will repay you, though I neither intend to do so, nor am I able to. I think I am somehow justified in lying to you because I really need the money. In such a situation, I would deliberately manipulate you to obtain a sum of money, thus using you as a means to my end. But this is morally impermissible as I have a direct duty to give you moral respect. Kant took the ground of such duties to be an objective quality possessed by people that is shared by all members of the moral community, and that is rationality. In other words, rationality is the quality that makes all rational beings morally important—to use Kant's language, it renders rational beings "ends-in-themselves." Thus, we are morally obligated by our rationality, for example, not to hurt other rational beings because, if we do, we hurt them directly by going against rationality.

Since animals are not rational beings by Kant's definition, we do not have direct duties to them; we cannot wrong them directly. However, cruel treatment of animals indirectly damages humanity. Consequently, we have *indirect* duties toward animals. Having indirect duties toward animals means that if I hurt or maltreat an animal, I do not hurt or maltreat the animal directly because animals lack reason; hence, I do not have any direct moral duty toward animals. Rather, according to the indirect duty view, I have certain duties about animals in the sense that by hurting them I unwittingly hurt humanity. That is to say, acting cruelly to animals may eventually lead to cruel actions toward rational beings. And since we have direct duties not to hurt rational beings, we should avoid cruelty to animals, which may trigger it.

My main contention here is that, to account for indirect duties to animals, the indirect duty view theorist must show that animals have some objective characteristic(s) by virtue of which our response to maltreating them translates into maltreating humans. But what could these characteristics be? It seems that if these characteristics exist, they need to be objective moral characteristics that cause all members of the moral community (all rational beings) to be affected by their treatment of rational beings as a result of their treatment of animals. But then it follows that animals have certain intrinsic moral features that make them ends-in-themselves. But by definition, animals are means and not ends. The question is, thus, if animals are mere means to our ends, why did Kant think that treating them well will make us better off morally toward other humans? What is the difference, then, between animals and, say, machines? Can we just as well say that treating machines well makes us treat each other with respect? Therefore, I argue that animals either have special moral characteristics or do not. If they do, then, contrary to the indirect duty view, we have a direct moral duty to them. If they do not, then we do not have any moral duty to them at all.[5]

KANT, MARGINAL CASES, AND ANIMALS

For Kant it is not possible to intelligibly assign obligations to beings who are incapable of making rules about what they ought to do and how to act on those rules, as described above. Thus this peculiar psychological capacity to freely construct the kind of moral legislation I described here is what defines humans as rational beings. Therefore, morality is for Kant the activity performed by free, rational agents of making laws—creating universal maxims to benefit all rational beings. Morality does not rest upon human-independent moral values, but rather on rationality.

It follows that animals, small children, and the severely mentally disabled (often referred to as marginal cases) are incapable of formulating categorical imperatives; consequently, moral duty does not apply to them directly in that rational beings have no duty to respect or foster the ends of marginal cases. However, according to Kant we cannot just do to them whatever we please. Specifically regarding animals, Kant argues, "If he is not to stifle his own feelings, he must practice kindness towards animals, for he who is cruel to animals becomes hard also in his dealings with men. We can judge the heart of a man by his treatment of animals."[6] It appears quite clear that Kant regarded those beings that lack rationality as mere things. Animals, as far as Kant was concerned, are things. However, it does not follow that we are permitted to mistreat them. The reason Kant gave for this is interesting. Kant was not worried that mistreatment of an animal wrongs the animal. Rather, he argued that one who is cruel to animals becomes cruel to humans. Thus, it is in the self-interest of humanity to treat animals kindly. In other words, our duties to animals are indirect and derive from our duty to respect and foster the ends of humanity. Our treatment of animals can be seemingly cruel only in the case that that treatment benefits humanity. Kant's view was that we should refrain from *pointless* cruelty to animals. Since animals' existence is solely to serve man, causing animal suffering is justified whenever it suits our interests. For example, he writes, "Vivisectionists, who use living animals for their experiments, certainly act cruelly, although their aim is praiseworthy, and they can justify their cruelty, since animals must be regarded as man's instruments; but any such cruelty for sport cannot be justified."[7] Note that here Kant recognized that animals do suffer. This distinguishes him from those who believe that animals are unfeeling automata. Still, Kant's ethical system, unlike utilitarianism, for example, is not concerned about suffering, but rather about duty and rationality. Humans, for Kant, are rational beings, and as such are ends-in-themselves; humans, for Kant, are the locus of morality by virtue of being rational. Conversely, animals, not being rational, are not intrinsically valuable. Animals lack the kind of rationality required to legislate and enforce moral laws. All of this means that we have a duty to respect other rational beings and treat them never as means to our ends, but always as ends-in-themselves. Since animals lack rationality, we are under no obligation to respect them; they are not ends-in-themselves, but rather means to our ends. Yet, according to Kant, it does not follow that we may do to animals anything we want. According to Kant, we have indirect duty toward animals. Our duty is indirect in at least two respects. First, animals often belong to some rational beings. Thus, maltreating or disrespecting those animals will ultimately wrong their owners. Second, Kant argues that acting cruelly toward animals affects negatively our treatment of other rational beings. This is a very interesting aspect of Kant's indirect duty principle. It suggests that as a matter of preventing possible emulation of cruelty toward other rational beings, we should refrain from maltreating animals.

WHAT'S WRONG WITH THE INDIRECT DUTY VIEW?

The principle of indirect duty implies that cruelty toward animals is not wrong in itself. It seems that Kant was not worried about cruelty itself; rather, he was concerned about misplacement of cruelty. He was concerned that maltreating animals can corrupt rational beings to the point that they might also treat other rational beings the same way. This view, however, strikes many as wrong, and for good reasons. If we are supposed to become better moral individuals and treat other humans with respect when we treat animals kindly, or, if our maltreating animals may cause us to maltreat other rational beings, Kant should give us a strong justification that such a causal relation exists. What if we were to treat animals badly and we treated humans kindly as a result? After all, Kant is clear about the moral status of animals: They are things and have no intrinsic moral worth. And if this is evident, then it does not seem hard to imagine that people could maltreat animals and as a result be kind to humans. The above quotations are very clear. Animals are like things. We do not have any moral duty to them. But if we have no moral obligations to treat animals with kindness, in principle we could do anything we want to them.[8] However, we refrain from doing so because, Kant tells us, by damaging an animal we harm humanity and ourselves. Animals, apparently for Kant, are objects that we can use to develop our kindness toward other humans: "He must practice kindness towards animals, for he who is cruel to animals becomes hard also in his dealings with men."[9] David DeGrazia points out that Kant's indirect duty view "does not hold up under careful scrutiny."[10] DeGrazia mentions that Robert Nozick also argues that Kant's view is wrong. In a long passage referring to the principle by Kant that cruelty to animals may promote a disposition to cruelty toward humans, Nozick writes that it is not true that such a "spillover" exists.

Why should we assume that a spillover exists? After all, Kant's moral agent is a free-willed rational being; it seems that by virtue of being rational and free, one should understand the difference between the treatment of things and the treatment of persons—that is, between animals and rational beings. A rational individual, then, as Kant describes it, should be able to recognize the moral distinctness of mere things and of rational individuals. And provided that he understands this difference, there is no reason to worry about a spillover. That is to say, I can understand the wrongness of hitting a rational person with a baseball bat because I am rational and value myself and do not intend that this type of act be done by anybody to anyone else (the universalizability principle). And if the other person is rational too, it is morally wrong to hit him with a bat. But by virtue of reason, I understand that animals are not rational and cannot reason like me. Also, following Kant's principle, animals are things—means to our ends. So I understand that hitting an animal with a bat is just like tearing up a piece of paper and, unless it belongs to someone else, I do not wrong the piece of paper if I tear it up—similarly, I do not wrong the animal if I beat it up. My being rational allows me to know that if I decide to beat an animal, I do so because the animal has no moral value. But I also know that I cannot cause pain to people because they are rational beings.

One of the problems with the indirect duty view is that, accordingly, our duty is not toward animals for their own sake, but rather for our own sake—the sake of humanity. The supposed purpose of indirect duty is to prevent our moral sensibility from being negatively affected by our treatment of animals because cruel treatment of animals may eventually mirror our treatment of humans. But if all it takes is for our treatment of humans not to be morally affected by our interaction with animals, in principle all rational beings could learn to be kind toward humans despite being cruel to animals; such a scenario is not hard to imagine. Then, according to the indirect duty view, at that point we would have no obligation toward animals, direct or indirect.

There is a problem with the indirect duty view that pertains to the causal connection between treating humans cruelly as a result of maltreating animals. Namely, indirect duty views suggest a causal connection between the way we treat animals and the attitude toward humans that results from our treatment of animals, such that if we wrong animals we are likely to do the same to humans. Kant believed this connection is founded on an analogy. Lara Denis, for example, endorses this view. She argues that what motivates us to treat animals kindly (according to the indirect duty view) is "certain analogies" between human behavior toward humans and animal behavior toward other animals and human-animal behavior. These analogies, she writes, "are such that we sometimes perceive animals' actions as following the same principles as our own."[11] For example, monkeys have been observed to mourn their dead, or bonobos to shake their heads to say no. Thus, although animals are only things and not persons, they have certain qualities that are analogous to human qualities.

However, what does this mean? How important are these qualities to establish the causal connection in question? Perhaps animals' behavior is analogous to ours, but it might only appear that way. What is important is that Kant never claims that certain animal behavior constitutes anything like a faculty of reason, which is the requirement for moral consideration. Despite certain similarities in behavior, according to Kant, animals are still things, and therefore we do not have direct duties toward them. Most importantly, these analogies between animal-animal and human-human and animal-human do not constitute a necessary causal connection, for reasons analogous to those listed in the previous paragraph. Essentially, Kant's position is at best a speculative psychological claim about human nature—that cruel treatment of animals makes people cold toward other people—which, even if he could prove it, is irrelevant because it is a contingent cultural fact about some human beings and not an objective fact about all rational beings. For, as I said, one can imagine people who were cruel to animals but never failed in their moral duties to humans. Gladly, bullfighting was banned in the Spanish community of Catalonia by a vote of the Catalan Parliament in July 2010. However, during the time that bullfighting was permitted, it does not seem that the cruelty inflicted upon the bulls created a spillover. After all, if what counts for a being to be fully considered a member of the moral community is rationality, and according to Kant animals lack rationality, that is all we need in order to know how to treat an animal. Namely, animals are merely things. And if they do not belong to other humans, we can treat them any way we like. It is not hard, in fact, to imagine rational beings able to make this kind of judgment, as a result of which they would torture animals but refrain from adopting such a behavior toward humans.

In other words, while some people might be psychologically moved by the behavior of animals such that their behavior toward humans might be affected, it does not follow that all rational beings would have the same reaction. In fact, what seems to be evident is that many people inflict gratuitous pain on animals but nevertheless respect other humans. Thus, there does not seem to be an objective, verifiable, and necessary connection between maltreating animals and transferring maltreatment to humans. As a side remark, there is a sense in which Kant's indirect duty view smacks of utilitarianism. Namely, since Kant is concerned about the possibility that those who are cruel to animals become hard also in their dealings with other rational beings,[12] it seems to me that Kant was worried about the repercussions of our actions upon others—in other words, he was concerned about the consequences of our actions. And if that is the case, it would seem a peculiarly consequentialist aspect of Kant's theory. Consequently, the indirect duty view fails to show that we have indirect duties to animals.

Kant refers to the mistaken notion that we have duties to animals as an amphiboly of the moral concepts of reflection.[13] With regard to ethics, Kant defines amphiboly as "taking what is a human being's duty to himself for a duty to other beings."[14] This means that any feeling of obligation that humans have toward animals rests upon a logical error. But if it is an error that leads us to take a human duty for a duty toward animals, and if it is this psychological connection that leads one to be cruel to humans when he is cruel to animals, then the solution is to train ourselves not to make that error. But again, this means that if we could train ourselves so that cruel treatment of animals never translates into cruel treatment of humans, then we would be morally warranted by Kant to perpetrate all sorts of hideousness upon animals because, as Kant points out, animals, like things, are not rational, and consequently are a mere means to our ends. Kant never claims that we ought not to use animals as mere means. Rather, he claims that we ought not to maltreat them. Given Kant's principle, we can use an animal as a means without maltreating it, as when, for example, a dog is used by the police to intercept explosives or drugs. But what does it mean to maltreat a thing? This is a misnomer. For, if I own a doll and pierce its eyes with a screwdriver, am I maltreating it? I do not think anyone would say that I am. But then, if I do the same to an animal, which, according to Kant is still a thing, why am I maltreating it? My point is that to say that something can be maltreated implies that something can be treated with cruelty, maltreated in a moral sense. In other words, it suggests that the subject being maltreated has an intrinsic moral value.

Moreover, Kant fails to provide an objective reason capable of grounding the assertion that cruelty to animals translates into cruel behavior toward humans. Our emotions or sympathy or our understanding of gratuitous cruelty is not enough to establish indirect duties toward animals. Kant's view shows that only certain people would be moved to have indirect duties toward animals—only those who recognize certain analogies between animals and humans and those who are duped by a moral amphiboly and believe that ill treatment of animals causes ill treatment of people. Other people who do not hold the same belief—people who are capable of rationally separating the way they treat animals and the way they treat humans (and understand the difference between the two)—could continue treating animals in any kind of way they please without worrying about duties. For, after all, if it can be guaranteed that one who treats animals cruelly nonetheless treats humans with respect, then he need only worry about direct duties toward humans and not indirect duties to things.

In order to show that we have indirect duties to animals, these duties should be universally applicable; but that means that one must provide objective grounds for them, showing that animals possess some objective characteristic or characteristics that generate a moral response in the form of indirect duty. Kant does a great job showing why we humans have *direct* duties toward other humans; namely, we possess something special, something objective, upon which we base moral values—and that is rationality. Humans are rational, but animals are not. Consequently, we have direct duties only toward humans—that is, rational beings. But he fails to show that there is a universal, objective trait or characteristic about animals capable of inclining us to behave cruelly toward humans were we to be cruel to animals. Kant could offer some objective reason for this connection only at the cost of undermining his indirect duty principle. He would have to say that animals possess something special that elicits in us a kind of response whereby cruelty to them makes us cruel to humans. This quality would have to be objective—for example, the capacity of suffering or some other objective quality to which all rational beings react.

Therefore, in the absence of some empirical evidence that animals have certain objective characteristics capable of justifying a moral response by all rational beings, we have no reason to believe that we have indirect duties toward animals. Unless and until Kantian ethicists provide evidence of such objective quality that animals possess, animals are, according to Kantian ethics, mere things that exist only for our benefit. However, in the event that one could point to such a trait possessed by animals, our duty toward animals would be direct, grounded in that particular trait. As it stands, Kant's moral system cannot account for either direct or indirect duties to animals.

TWO NEO-KANTIAN VIEWS

Here I would like to discuss two important deontological views that differ from Kant's in that animals have inherent moral value. The views that I discuss in what follows are those of Christine Korsgaard and Tom Regan. Korsgaard and Regan, unlike Kant, argue that animals do have intrinsic moral value, and consequently we have a duty to respect them. Korsgaard appeals to the notion that animals, like humans, are ends-in-themselves insofar as wronging them involves wronging their animal nature. After all, maltreating a person is a violation of his or her rational nature, as Kant argued, but in an important sense, maltreating others is wrong because it attacks their animal nature; namely, abusing causes physical suffering. Thus, animal nature for Korsgaard is one of the factors by virtue of which animals are intrinsically valuable. Regan also argues that the correct approach is to regard animals as intrinsically valuable. However, he does not specify exactly what factor or factors confer moral importance upon animals. Rather, Regan argues for animals' inherent value in negative terms.[15] Namely, he argues that regarding individuals as valuable according to certain characteristics is wrong. Utilitarians regard the individual as having no intrinsic moral value. The value is the aggregate happiness or satisfaction of preference for the greatest number of beings. This principle, according to Regan, leads to absurd implications (some of which I will discuss in the next section)—for example, that killing an innocent person might be permissible provided that doing so will lead to the greatest amount of happiness for the greatest number of beings. Regan points out that we should reject a perfectionist theory according to which moral values depend on certain characteristics, such as intelligence, the capacity to reason, and so on. Thus, he concludes that all animals that are subjects-of-a-life are intrinsically valuable. By the term "subject-of-a-life" Regan refers to all creatures whose life can be good or bad for them—that is, with respect to the kind of creatures they are. Thus Regan seems to just assume, without providing evidence, that all subjects-of-a-life have equal inherent value. And based on this assumption, Regan argues his case for animal rights.

To start with Korsgaard, in her lecture "Fellow Creatures: Kantian Ethics and Our Duties to Animals," she offers a revisionary reading of Kant with the intent to show how Kantian ethics can grant moral duties toward animals. She seems to imply that Kant was not consistent with his principles and made an error in his assessment of our duties toward animals. And if he had been consistent, he would have realized that animals are in a sense ends-in-themselves, and thus we have direct moral duties to them. Many Kantian ethicists have attempted to show that Kant's ethical system allows direct duties to animals. But have they succeeded? I think not. The problem is that Kant's ethical system is rather strict, because accordingly, only beings that have a rational nature can constrain us morally. By rational nature, according to Korsgaard, Kant refers to "our capacity to govern ourselves by autonomous rational choice."[16] Humans are rational creatures who form what Kant calls the "Kingdom of Ends." In the Kingdom of Ends, each individual is autonomous and capable of creating and understanding moral laws. Consequently, we humans have a duty to treat all members of our kingdom with respect. It is interesting to note that Kant believes that any kind of beings—human or Martians—endowed with a rational nature are part of the moral community. Unfortunately for animals, according to Kant, they are not moral agents because they are not rational in a way that they could ever govern themselves by autonomous rational choice; in terms of Kantian ethics, this means that we do not owe moral duties to animals—at least not directly. It is true that Kant concedes that we should be nice to animals so that we foster the right attitude toward the members of the Kingdom of Ends. But essentially we have no direct duties toward animals and are morally justified in killing them, eating them, and wearing them, but without violence or cruelty because it is demeaning to ourselves. In other words, so long as we have a sound justification, Kant's theory allows us to regard animals as property.

Kant's view, as Korsgaard points out, is an argument "from the capacity to obligate, or the lack of that capacity, to the assignment of a certain kind of value."[17] In other words, Kant does not want to say that animals have no value at all, but rather that they are not capable of obligating us to respect moral laws. Animals cannot enforce upon us moral obligations. And the question is whether animals are in fact capable of placing us under moral obligations; Korsgaard thinks that they are, though it appears to be the contrary. Korsgaard's thesis is that "despite appearances, and despite what he himself thought, Kant's argument reveals the ground of our obligations to the other animals."[18]

Korsgaard argues that Kant conflates two conceptions of "end-in-itself." One is the source of normative claims recognized by all rational agents. And the other sense is someone who is able to give force to a claim by participation in morality. Surely animals cannot be ends-in-themselves in the second sense because they lack rationality and autonomy; they do not participate in morality. But it does not follow that non-human animals cannot be ends-in-themselves in the first sense: as the sources of normative claims. It does not follow, Korsgaard says, that "there is no sense in which they can obligate us."[19] There *is*, in fact, a sense in which animals obligate us.

We take ourselves and our interests to be the source of morality. But we do not value our interests *only* because they are the interests of autonomous rational beings. Being autonomous and rational allows me to legislate against what is bad for me and others like me. However, I do not legislate, for example, against being lied to, being injured, being cheated on, etc., *only* because I am an autonomous and a rational being, but also—perhaps most importantly—because bad things assault my animal nature. In other words, "we object to pain and torture or injury because they are bad for us as animal beings."[20] In fact, Kant holds that respect for our rational nature involves respecting our animal nature. This is the ground for his arguments about our duties to ourselves, our self-preservation, the enjoyment of food, and sex. In the *Metaphysics of Morals* we find a section titled "A Human Being's Duty to Himself as an Animal Being."[21] Here Kant discusses duties to ourselves as animal beings with respect to our animal nature, not duties. He covers the duties not to commit suicide, not to maim or disfigure oneself, not to masturbate, and not to indulge in excessive use of food or drinks. Also, in *Religion within the Boundaries of Mere Reason*, Kant argues that our animal nature is one of three "original predispositions to good in human nature."[22]

> All these predispositions in the human being are not only (negatively) good (they do not resist the moral law) but they are also predispositions to the good (they demand compliance with it). They are original, for they belong to the possibility of human nature. The human being can indeed use the first two inappropriately, but cannot eradicate either of the two.[23]

Thus, Korsgaard concludes, animal nature is an end-in-itself, and that is why we have direct duties to non-human animals as well. In other words, for Korsgaard our autonomous nature is not the only source of normative claims. Besides our autonomous nature, we derive moral, normative value from our animal nature.

The duties we owe to ourselves arise out of the natural fact that many things can be objectively good or bad for us—for example, pain and suffering. Thus, while it is true that animals are not self-legislative beings capable of imposing laws upon us, it does not follow that we owe no moral duties directly to them at all. In fact, animals, like us, are beings for whom things can be good or bad. So, Kant is mistaken because he does not recognize this. As Korsgaard puts it, "human incentives are simply the same as those of the other animals."[24] And she also reminds us that Kant does not believe that humans are magnificently unique in the sense that their nature is transcendental, unlike animals.[25] Humans are not morally superior in this sense for Kant. Rather, humans are able to legislate that the things that are good for us are the source of normative claims. This is certainly one sense in which humans are ends-in-themselves; the other sense is that they have an animal nature. Thus, animal nature is an end-in-itself—and it follows that we have direct duties to other animals.

Korsgaard's reevaluation of Kant's indirect duty view is an interesting attempt to redeem Kant's moral view on animals. Korsgaard implies that today we know a great deal more about animals and animal minds that Kant arguably was not aware of, although her main revision of Kant doesn't turn on any knowledge about animals that Kant didn't have. Our knowledge has allowed us to recognize that many animals are, to use Kant's terminology, ends-in-themselves. In other words, she argues that Kant should have recognized on his own principle that we have direct duties to animals because direct duties are grounded in animal nature. For Korsgaard, Kant was wrong about claiming that only rational beings can place us under moral obligation, but I doubt that Korsgaard's attempt is successful. Korsgaard's success in showing that we have direct duties to animals on a Kantian ground hinges on the question of whether Kant in fact overlooked the implications of his own principle. Or to put it simply, would Kant agree with Korsgaard's characterization of his moral view about animals? I do not think it is clear that Kant would concede that having an animal nature is morally important because when we legislate against things that assault us, we in fact make laws against them because they assault our animal nature. Having an animal nature may be a sufficient condition for having direct duties to other rational beings but not a necessary condition. That is to say, our animal nature is, after all, "attached" to—comes with—a rational nature, but animals (according to Kant) are completely devoid of a rational nature—and that is why they cannot put us under moral obligation (i.e., we do not have direct moral duties to them).

Korsgaard's account of Kant's indirect duty to animals could, nonetheless, be championed to defend animals. But at what cost? As I pointed out, there is no clear textual evidence that Kant overlooked the possibility that animal nature can be a source of normativity. Furthermore, there is no textual evidence that Kant would regard animal nature alone as important enough to consider animals as ends-in-themselves. What, in the end, Korsgaard's conclusion provides is an account that disassociates itself from the Kantian tradition and, strangely, shares certain views—for example, the fact that we should consider that animals suffer—with utilitarian ethics. But even if Korsgaard is successful in showing that Kant's moral theory has the resources to grant that we have direct moral duties to animals, her theory does not move us in the direction of respecting animals—just as Kant's theory fails to do so. Korsgaard is seriously interested in the issue of our treatment of animals and wants to offer moral grounds for treating animals with respect; but her proposed approach won't do any good. Even if, according to her revisionary version of Kant's view, it turns out that we have direct moral duties toward animals, such duties won't guarantee that animals will not be eaten or used as subjects of scientific research. After all, Kant himself was not against using animals as a source of food and as subjects for scientific research, provided this was necessary and we inflicted no gratuitous cruelty upon animals. And it is not accidental that Korsgaard is not defending veganism and does not explicitly condemn the use of animals for food. She is a vegetarian. Her proposed moral approach presents the same limitations as Kant's: It focuses on duty and says nothing about the importance of having a good moral character.

What this means is that in her view, it is possible to respect animals while using them and their by-products. The account that she champions is consistent with an attitude that regards animals as creatures that have interests, a life, and existence, and these factors oblige us to respect animals. But it is perfectly consistent, morally acceptable, on Korsgaard's account, to use animals and their by-products so long as those animals are not offended or hurt. The view that I propose here is that of veganism as a virtuous attitude toward animals—that is, the idea that animals have an intrinsic moral value and as such they ought not to be used as sources of food. This view, I believe, is consistent with an understanding that animals are not our property.

This last consideration brings me to a second point that, even if it is successful, Korsgaard's reinterpretation of Kant's view on our duties toward animals fails as a moral theory in favor of animals because her view is ultimately concerned with notions of obligation and right conduct. The problem is the very conception of morality as a set of universal and authoritative norms that all moral agents are categorically obligated to follow. My position is that this conception of morality is defective. Deontology tells us to view the world from an individual point of view, but morality, in my view, is about how we treat others, not about ourselves and how we use our individual reflections to derive categorically imperative norms. To end this section, I want to reflect upon a serious criticism of the kind of moral outlook proposed by Korsgaard. Korsgaard argues, "Morality assigns us purposes, it is our moral duty to help those in need for its own sake—not to help those in need for something else. We are creatures who adopt our purposes—they are not given to us by our desires, and that means we need principles to guide their adoption."[26] To show why Korsgaard's moral outlook about our treatment of animals fails, I want to consider Michael Stocker's criticism of duty-based theories. Stocker goes directly to the heart of the problem as he writes,

> These theories [referring to Kantian and utilitarian ethics] are, thus, doubly defective. As ethical theories, they fail by making it impossible for a person to achieve the good in an integrated way. As theories of the mind, of reasons and motives, of human life and activity, they fail, not only by putting us in a position that is psychologically uncomfortable, difficult, or even untenable, but also by making us and our lives essentially fragmented and incoherent.[27]

As Stocker points out, a theory that emphasizes duty leads us to moral schizophrenia. That is to say, imagine that you are in a hospital, recovering from an illness. Your friend comes in to visit you, and this makes you happy. However, you find out that he is unenthusiastic about visiting you. In fact, he would rather be somewhere else. He came to see you not because he loves you and he is concerned about your health, but rather because he is a deontologist who is committed to acting out of duty, regardless of how he feels about a certain action. Now think what this moral outlook comes to when applied to the treatment of animals. Such a moral view asks us to respect animals because we should recognize that we have certain moral duties toward them. The trouble is that many people tend to agree with Kant when it comes to our relationship with animals—namely, they are not rational creatures, so we are justified in killing and eating them.

Tom Regan's approach is another example of deontological ethics. Regan proposes a strong animal rights position, the view that animals have the same basic moral rights as humans. To be clear, Regan does not argue that animals should have exactly the same rights that human beings have, such as voting, obtaining a driver's license, buying a house, or getting married. Rather, all animals have a right to life and consequently should not be used for food. Therefore, we should all be vegans. In addition to this, animals should not be used as subjects for scientific research, entertainment, hunting, etc. As Regan argues,

> The fundamental wrong is the system that allows us to view animals as *our resources*, here for *us*—to be eaten, or surgically manipulated, or exploited for sport or money. Once we accept this view of animals—as our resources—the rest is as predictable as it is regrettable.[28]

In *The Case for Animal Rights* Regan argues that all mammals, including cows, pigs, and goats (those mammals that are typically eaten by people), over a year of age have the same basic moral rights as humans. Regan presents his argument, as Mary Anne Warren points out,[29] in three stages. The first stage is to note that animals, such as those I just mentioned, are more than mere fleshy machines, as Descartes believed. Animals are sentient creatures, but more importantly, they have memory, emotions, desires, identity over time, and other important mental characteristics that are relevantly similar to those possessed by humans. Consequently, Regan believes that animals that possess such capacities are subjects-of-a-life. And since subjects-of-a-life can be harmed or benefited, it follows that animals can be harmed or benefited. Therefore, animals have a right not to be harmed and we have a duty to respect that right—just like we ought to respect basic human rights. Here I find myself in agreement with Regan.

The second stage, however, is more problematic. Regan argues that subjects-of-a-life have inherent value. While Kant, as we have seen, argued that animals are mere means to our ends, Regan argues that since animals are subjects-of-a-life, they are ends-in-themselves. According to Regan, all animals have inherent value—that is, inherent value does not come in degrees. To say that some animals have more value than others, according to Regan, is to adopt a perfectionist moral view, which assigns different moral value on the basis of certain characteristics—for example, intelligence, species, etc. We know from history that such a theory could justify many unjust positions, such as slavery, male domination, racism, etc. Thus, Regan argues that we must reject the perfectionist view and adopt a view according to which we divide all living things into two categories: those that have inherent value, which have the same basic rights as humans, and those that do not have inherent moral value, which have no moral right. Consequently, all subjects-of-a-life must be regarded as having rights.

The third stage is to argue that all beings that have an inherent moral value must be respected; they must not be treated as mere means to our ends. This implies that we have a direct prima facie duty to respect and avoid harming all subjects-of-a-life. It is these considerations that generate moral rights. All morally valuable beings have a right to life. And rights imply obligations. We have the duty to avoid harming others or treating them as means to our ends—moreover we have the duty to avoid harm and help others that are endangered.

While I find many points of agreement with Regan's argument, I am dubious of the soundness of such an argument. I will briefly explain some difficulties. Regan places a great deal of importance on the distinction between normal mature mammals and other species. In his defense, perhaps Regan wanted to emphasize normal mammals for practical reasons: firstly, animal agriculture treats normal mammals horribly. Thus, Regan wanted to discuss the imminent problem, one that seems very clear-cut. Secondly, Regan might have thought that if we accept his argument, a great deal of injustice and animal suffering could be avoided since they are mainly caused by animal agriculture. Perhaps Regan thought that if we accept his subject-of-a-life principle, we will eventually be kind and considerate to all forms of life and even the environment. However, his emphasis on normal mammals generates difficulties. For example, what makes a mammal more special than a reptile or a bird? And why does the animal have to be a normal mature one to have inherent value? I find it peculiar that Regan proposes that there should be any correlation between age and inherent value when his very theory argues that inherent moral value does not come in degrees. One possible answer is that whenever we are uncertain of whether a being is a subject-of-a-life, we may give it the benefit of the doubt. However, how exactly is it to be applied? As Warren notes,

> But if we try to apply this principle to the entire range of doubtful cases, we will find ourselves with moral obligations which we cannot possibly fulfill. In many climates, it is virtually impossible to live without swatting mosquitoes and exterminating cockroaches, and not all of us can afford to hire someone to sweep the path before we walk, in order to make sure that we do not step on ants.[30]

Indeed, according to Regan's argument, since animals, like humans, have a life that can go well or can be frustrated, they all have the right to life and to be treated with respect. But it does not seem to follow from this that every life has the same value. Is it true that animals have the same value as humans? Granted, Regan states a qualification: that animals have a life that, like humans, can go well or badly *for them*. If a squirrel has a good life, it depends on factors that are different from the factors that make a human life good. However, does it follow that squirrels and humans should have the same basic rights? Speaking of squirrels, James Rachels used a Lockean characterization of the right of property to conclude that

> If Locke is right, then it follows that animals such as squirrels also have a right to property; for squirrels labor to gather nuts for their own nourishment in exactly the way Locke pictures the man laboring. There is no relevant difference between the man and the squirrel: they both pick up the nuts, take them home, store them away, and then eat them. Therefore there is no justification for saying that the man has a right to the nuts he gathers, but that the squirrel does not.[31]

However, the very concept of right, especially human rights, is not an uncontroversial one. At any rate, Rachels here makes an unwarranted jump from the principle of human rights (which is itself controversial) to the conclusion that squirrels also have rights in the same respect as humans. But humans, if anything, have rights by virtue of the fact that they have an understanding of rights and they can enforce them upon others. As Carl Cohen stated,

> This much is clear about rights in general: they are in every case claims, or potential claims, within a community of moral agents. Rights arise, and can be intelligently defended, only among beings who actually do, or can, make moral claims against one another.[32]

I must say that the first time I read Regan's *The Case for Animal Rights*, I found many ideas that resonated with me. Regan's is an admirable position for promoting ethical veganism. However, his argument is not conducive to respect of animals because it is unpersuasive. And it is unpersuasive because it is based on wrong assumptions. The overall issues with such an argument are the idea that because animals, like humans, have a life that can be good or bad *for them*, it follows that both humans and animals have the same basic rights. This does not seem to follow if we consider that talking about rights, as many have pointed out, makes sense in a context in which the parties can intelligently make sense and impose certain rights. Animals, obviously, would be excluded. Furthermore, Regan's approach to the question of our treatment of animals is, after all, a deontological view, and thus suffers from the same criticisms that apply to Kantian and neo-Kantian theories. That is, our moral obligations toward others should not be an all-or-nothing affair. A viable animal ethics theory, in my view, should be flexible enough to account for exceptions and account for the particularities of circumstances. Moreover, a viable approach is one that is internally motivating. In other words, one could easily agree with Regan, with the notion of rights; however, there is a gap between the acceptance of a logical argument (provided that the argument is sound) and acting accordingly. What could possibly bridge that gap? What could motivate one to be against all forms of animal exploitation? The acceptance of Regan's argument, therefore, is not conducive to respecting animals.

Such a theory of supposed duties is neither able to convince many, nor to motivate those who might be convinced! It appears clear that Kantianism (or neo-Kantianism) is not a viable moral theory capable of making sense of the morality of our relation with animals; it is not a theory that can be used to defend the interests of animals.

NOTES

1. Nicholas Wademarch, "Scientist Finds the Beginnings of Morality in Primate Behavior," *New York Times*, March 20, 2007. http://www.nytimes.com/2007/03/20/science/20moral.html.
2. Immanuel Kant, *Lectures on Ethics*, trans. Louis Infield (New York: Harper & Row, 1963), 24.
3. Ibid., 239–241.
4. Immanuel Kant, *Lectures on Anthropology* 7, 127.
5. As I will indicate later, Robert Nozik and David DeGrazia have brought up this objection. But others have made similar points: See, for example, Alice Crary, "What Already Matters: A Critique of Moral Individualism," *Philosophical Topics* 38, no. 1 (Spring 2010): 17–49; and Allen W. Wood, "Kant on Duties Regarding Nonrational Nature," *Proceedings of the Aristotelian Society, Supplementary Volumes* 72 (1998): 189–228.
6. Kant, *Lectures on Ethics*, 212 (27: 459).
7. Kant, *Lecture on Ethics*, 239.
8. But Kant is not a consequentialist!
9. Kant, *Lectures on Ethics*, 212 (27: 459).
10. David DeGrazia, *Taking Animals Seriously* (Cambridge: Cambridge University Press, 1996), 42.
11. Lara Denis, "Kant's Conception of Duties regarding Animals: Reconstruction and Reconsideration," *History of Philosophy Quarterly* 17, no. 4 (October 2000): 405–423.
12. Kant, *Lectures on Ethics*, 212 (27: 459).
13. Immanuel Kant, *The Metaphysics of Morals*, in *Practical Philosophy*, ed. and trans. M. J. Gregor (Cambridge: Cambridge University Press, 1999), 353–603.
14. Kant, *The Metaphysics of Morals*, 6:422.
15. Mary Anne Warren, "Difficulties with the Strong Animal Rights Position," *Between the Species* 2, no. 4 (1986): 347.
16. Christine Korsgaard, "Fellow Creatures: Kantian Ethics and Our Duties to Animals," in *The Tanner Lectures on Human Values*, ed. G. B. Peterson (Salt Lake City, 2005), 3.
17. Korsgaard, "Fellow Creatures," 16–17.
18. Ibid., 5.
19. Ibid., 21.
20. Ibid., 28.
21. Immanuel Kant, *Metaphysics of Morals*.
22. Kant, *Religion*, 6:28, 74.
23. Ibid., 6:28, 76.
24. Korsgaard, "Fellow Creatures," 32.
25. Ibid., 33.

26. Korsgaard, cited in Katrien Schaubroeck, "Interview with Christine Korsgaard, Holder of the Cardinal Mercier Chair 2009," *The Leuven Philosophy Newsletter* 17 (2008–2009/2009–2010): 55.

27. Michael Stocker, "The Schizophrenia of Modern Moral Theories," *Journal of Philosophy* 73 (1976): 455.

28. In Peter Singer, ed., *In Defense of Animals* (New York: Basil Blackwell, 1985), 13.

29. Warren, "Difficulties with the Strong Animal Rights Position," 346.

30. Warren, 348.

31. In Tom Regan and Peter Singer, eds., *Animal Rights and Human Obligations* (Englewood Cliffs: Prentice-Hall, 1989), 206.

32. Carl Cohen, "The Case for the Use of Animals in Biomedical Research," *The New England Journal of Medicine* 315 (1986): 865.

Chapter Two

Utilitarianism

All That Is Gold Does Not Glitter

SOME BASIC TENETS OF UTILITARIANISM

Having considered Kant and neo-Kantians' moral principles, I shall now consider another important moral theory: utilitarianism. Utilitarianism is a form of teleological ethics, because it argues that what is ultimately important in morality are the consequences of our actions. More specifically, utilitarians argue that what makes an action good or right is measured on the basis of how much happiness or pleasure a particular action can produce: an action is deemed good just if its consequences promote the maximal amount of happiness for the greatest number of beings; an action is bad just if its consequences lead to a prevalence of unhappiness over happiness. Utilitarianism is an attractive moral theory for good reasons. To mention one, it is an egalitarian approach to morality. What's morally important is not rationality or race or language skills or any other characteristics of this nature. Utilitarianism does not even discriminate against a particular species. Every moral theory has a specific starting point. Deontology starts with rationality, and religious morality starts with the goodness of God, while utilitarianism starts with sentience. Sentience, the capacity to experience pain and pleasure, is the locus or ground of morality. Contra Kant, animals (though not all) are also morally important because they possess the capacity to feel pain or pleasure—that is, they are sentient beings. Not surprisingly, utilitarians have been fervent proponents of animal rights and vegetarianism.[1]

The concept of utilitarianism has its origin in Epicureanism. However, the works of Jeremy Bentham (1748–1842), John Stuart Mill (1806–1873), and Henry Sidgwick (1838–1900) popularized utilitarianism. Jeremy Bentham,

John Stuart Mill, and Henry Sidgwick argued for the moral importance of animals. They believed that the interests of animals should be respected just as much as those of humans. Bentham's utilitarianism is a hedonistic approach to morality according to which "the measure of right and wrong" is the greatest happiness of the greatest number. It was Bentham who wrote that in morality, "The question is not, Can they reason? nor, Can they talk? but, Can they suffer?"[2] By "happiness," Bentham refers to a predominance of pleasure over pain. As he writes in *The Principles of Morals and Legislation*,

> Nature has placed mankind under the governance of two sovereign masters, pain and pleasure. It is for them alone to point out what we ought to do, as well as to determine what we shall do. On the one hand the standard of right and wrong, on the other the chain of causes and effects, are fastened to their throne. They govern us in all we do, in all we say, in all we think.[3]

In other words, the goal of morality is to act in such ways that the outcomes of our actions should maximize happiness and minimize unhappiness for the greatest number. To determine which actions should be taken, Bentham suggested a procedure known as the hedonistic or felicific calculus. The calculus consists in a number of criteria that are used to determine the right action in a given situation. The criteria include, for example, the intensity, duration, certainty, proximity, and purity of happiness generated by a certain action.

John Stuart Mill adopted the main idea of Bentham's utilitarianism. Like Bentham, Mill argued that the maximal happiness of sentient beings is the goal of morality. Mill's hedonistic approach, however, is distinctive from Bentham's in that Mill gave particular importance to the ethical life of intellectual pleasures and to utilitarian rules. He noted that most people place greater importance upon intellectual pleasures, such as education, philosophical discussions, and art, over physical pleasures. Consequently, the attainment of happiness requires development of one's intellectual faculties.

Also, Mill's utilitarianism makes room for moral rules as utilitarian tools that are conducive to the greatest good for the greatest number. Mill argues that certain moral rules—for example, "Keep your promises" and "Tell the truth"—typically produce happiness and promote the welfare of society. This version of the theory is referred to as "rule utilitarianism." Normally we should follow these utilitarian rules without thinking too much about the consequences of our acts. However, such rules should be jettisoned in the event that they conflict with the maximization of utility.

Later, it was Australian philosopher Peter Singer who used a particular version of utilitarianism, known as "preference utilitarianism," which was initially outlined by Richard Mervyn Hare, to support the animal rights movement. In one of his most recent works Singer reveals that he has since become a hedonistic utilitarian because he finds the arguments in favor to be more persuasive than those in favor of preference utilitarianism.[4] Preference utilitarianism differs from that of Bentham and Mill. Essentially, Bentham and Mill argued that utility is pleasure or happiness, while according to preference utilitarianism utility is preference.[5] That is, for Mill and Bentham, a moral action is right if its consequences produce the greatest amount of pleasure or happiness for the greatest number of beings that have the capacity to feel pleasure and happiness. Preference utilitarianism takes the right action to be that which promotes the preferences of all sentient beings.[6] Although Singer recently changed his mind, he used his preference utilitarianism to show that humans have a moral obligation to stop raising animals for food and to stop using animals as subjects for scientific research. His main arguments can be found in the now very popular books *Animal Liberation* (1975) and *Practical Ethics* (1979). These two works, among others by Singer, played a vital role in shaping the contemporary animal rights movement and the philosophy of vegetarianism.

According to preference utilitarianism, the right action, rather than calculating pleasure against pain, is one that promotes the best interests of the greatest number of sentient beings. Accordingly, Singer argues that "applying the principle of utility to our present situation—especially the methods now used to rear animals for food and the variety of foods available to us—leads to the conclusion that we ought to be vegetarians."[7] But is it true that utilitarianism leads to that conclusion? In what follows, I want to show that utilitarianism is not a viable moral system to claim and support the rights of animals and does not lead necessarily to vegetarianism, that utilitarianism does not underwrite concern about the welfare of animals at all.

Perhaps it can be useful to understand utilitarianism by contrasting it with deontology. Deontology, as we have seen, says that the right moral action is one that is performed by a rational being in conformity with universally recognized rules. For a deontologist, the consequences of an action are irrelevant insofar as establishing which action is right; what counts are the reasons for performing a certain action. For example, suppose that lying in a particular circumstance might be more beneficial to a number of individuals than telling the truth. Deontology says that although it might be the case that lying is more beneficial, lying is wrong because it is irrational. A world where people are permitted to lie whenever seems convenient is irrational, thus immoral, and therefore one must always tell the truth. Contrariwise, for a utilitarian lying is not necessarily wrong in itself. Granted, rule utilitarians might object that truth telling is a utilitarian rule that more often than not produces the best result. However, it is not the only view of rule utilitarianism. Some rule utilitarians argue that utilitarian rules should be followed unless they clearly do not lead to the best result, in which case the rules need not be followed. Thus, in general, utilitarians emphasize the importance of the aggregate satisfaction rather than strictly following rules. For example, if

I save a man who is drowning in the Hudson River because I am promised a monetary reward and not because I think it is the right thing to do, according to utilitarianism I do the right thing. For utilitarianism it is not important why I perform an action, but rather the end result—not any end result, but one that generates the greatest good for the greatest number of beings. Utilitarianism's thesis is very simple: right actions are those that *in the long run* maximize utility and minimize disutility for the greatest number of sentient beings.[8] It follows that if I save a person from drowning and as a result that person is happy, his family and friends are happy, I am happy, the mayor is happy, and no one is unhappy or very few are unhappy, I have done the right thing; regardless of my motivation, I have done the right thing because I saved a life or, to put it in technical terms, I maximized aggregate utility.

In its traditional versions, utilitarianism sees utility as pleasure or happiness, and disutility as pain or suffering. Hence, right actions are those that in the long run promote the greatest happiness/pleasure for the greatest number of sentient beings. According to Singer's formerly endorsed version, maximizing utility involves a consideration of the preferences of all sentient beings involved. In other words, preference utilitarianism argues that right actions are those that produce consequences that best serve the interest, or that satisfy the preferences, of the greatest number of sentient beings. A statement that Singer makes in *Practical Ethics* adroitly captures his view:

> The way of thinking I have outlined is a form of utilitarianism. It differs from classical utilitarianism in that "best consequences" is understood as meaning what, on balance, furthers the interests of those affected, rather than merely what increases pleasure and reduces pain. (It has, however, been suggested that classical utilitarians like Bentham and John Stuart Mill used "pleasure" and "pain" in a broad sense that allowed them to include achieving what one desired as a "pleasure" and the reverse as a "pain").[9]

I used the term "sentient" a number of times because it is an important aspect of utilitarianism. Singer understands the term "sentience" to mean "the capacity for suffering and enjoying things."[10] This includes creatures like humans, cows, pigs, chickens, and all other creatures capable of feeling pain and pleasure. Consequently, humans as well as non-human animals deserve equal moral consideration in virtue of their capacity to experience pain/pleasure. While for Kant, as we saw earlier, rationality is the locus of morality, according to utilitarianism, sentience is the starting point of moral consideration, the special characteristic that confers upon a being moral worth. In the words of Singer,

> If a being suffers, there can be no moral justification for refusing to take that suffering into consideration. No matter what the nature of the being, the princi-

ple of equality requires that its suffering be counted equally with the like suffering—in so far as rough comparisons can be made—of any other being.[11]

The idea is that since animals are sentient beings, they have preferences— they prefer to live a life free of pain, and therefore their preferences should be given the same consideration that we give to the interests of humans. When we think about those animals whose body parts typically turn up on people's plates, such as cows, chickens, lambs, pigs, and fish, we realize that they can experience pleasure or pain. These animals are unlike rocks and very much like humans in that their life can be miserable or happy. Therefore, preference utilitarianism argues, acknowledging the fundamental fact that most animals are sentient, and that this capacity renders a being worthy of moral consideration, that we are obliged to avoid causing pain.

Considering animals' suffering and regarding the interests of animals as important, according to Singer, does not mean to say that animals may be, for example, sedated before being slaughtered or treated well while alive and then slaughtered and eaten.[12] Based on the principles of utilitarianism, it is not morally permissible to raise animals for food or to use animals for testing in scientific research. It has to be noted, however, that in Singer's view, and indeed in the view of utilitarians in general, being opposed to eating animals is relative to time and place. The salient nature of utilitarianism is to deny that there are absolute rules that we all must follow. Thus, given certain circumstances, but not all circumstances, vegetarianism promotes the greatest good for the greatest number of sentient beings. As Singer writes, "Whether we ought to be vegetarians depends on a lot of facts about the situation in which we find ourselves." And it also reminds us that he rejects "all these forms of moral absolutism."[13] Accordingly, killing and eating the flesh of animals, eating their eggs, and using animal by-products is not immoral as such, but rather depends upon the situation.[14] For example, in regions of the world where vegetables do not grow, due to hostile climatic conditions or other unfavorable factors, using animals as food would be morally permissible. But in affluent countries, where plant-based food is abundant and readily available, vegetarianism is the only logical conclusion.[15]

Singer argues that once we properly understand the idea of equal moral consideration, there is no reason to deny that sentient animals have interests that are equal to human interests.[16] When we consider what equality really means, we realize that eating animals stems from a latent form of prejudice, which he refers to as "speciesism." Speciesism is a form of racism toward other species, in the instant case sentient animals. The idea is that this prejudice is wrong because it implies that one group, in this case one species, claims to be morally superior to others. If we accept that prejudice toward a certain group or race or sex or gender is wrong, Singer argues, then we are mistaken in treating animals as property because we are guilty of speciesism—that is, we claim that human animals are morally superior to non-human animals, and consequently we may use animals for our benefit.

The interesting aspect of the moral approach proposed by Singer is that there are important differences among groups. After all, the argument typically goes, human beings are superior to animals. Look at what they do. They write poetry, build spacecrafts, and more. In other words, animals and humans are not equal. However, not all humans write poetry and build spacecrafts. Many individuals are not even capable of building paper airplanes. The fact that humans are unequal is precisely the reason that Singer suggests that moral consideration should be based on the capacity to experience pain/pleasure. Such capacity is the basis of all interests. A rock lacks interests. A mouse has them. Thus, for Singer the only possible way to discriminate individuals is a dichotomy between sentient and non-sentient beings. The pleasure that one experiences from eating meat is not a valid justification for using animals for food. That pleasure must be weighed against the suffering caused by humans to animals.

To sum up, preference utilitarianism offers a remarkable argument for vegetarianism: Individuals (humans and non-humans) are different. Some are smart and some are not, some are cute and some are ugly, some are strong and some are weak. But these characteristics are not morally relevant; they are mere subjective characteristics. In fact, if the ability to write poetry or to build spacecrafts renders one morally superior to others, then it would be bad news for most of us. Instead, what counts in morality is the objective fact that all sentient beings have the capacity to experience pain/pleasure, by virtue of which such beings have preferences. Therefore, the preference of all animals must be taken into consideration. And thus with regard to our duty toward animals, those who have easy access to plant-based food have the moral obligation to be or become vegetarians. The way we understand the preference principle is by considering the impact that the meat and dairy industry has on the environment, on the human body, and on the lives of animals. It turns out that raising animals for food has a tremendously negative impact on nature, our natural resources, and our health. In utilitarian terms this means that using animals for our food and other benefits generates more disutility than utility; or, to put it another way, using animals for food leads to the greatest amount of unhappiness for the greatest number of beings. This is obviously an unsatisfactory result since our actions for utilitarianism should promote the greatest amount of happiness for the greatest number of beings.

UTILITARIANISM = VEGETARIANISM?

Utilitarians offer a compelling argument for vegetarianism. However, I find that there is something fundamentally wrong with the utilitarian approach to animal ethics. Perhaps this extravagant analogy will help express my point. Utilitarianism reminds me of a joke. A biker, á la *Easy Rider*, travels with his inseparable companion dog. While on the road, they observe a moribund fawn. The biker's attitude appears to be very compassionate: he pulls over to tend to the fawn and then says, "I can't stand seeing you suffer." He then draws his handgun and shoots the wounded fawn dead. Another time, he notices a car accident where a driver is still alive but in very bad condition. Again, he takes his gun and, reciting the same line, puts the man out of his misery. One day the biker himself has the misfortune of being t-boned by an inattentive driver. Waking after a short time in an unconscious state, he realizes that he has a few bruises but is not badly hurt, and he rejoices at the sight of his dog friend also having survived the accident. But when he notices that his dog is bleeding profusely, he gropes for his handgun and says, "I can't stand seeing you suffer." And just as he is about to pull the trigger, his dog shouts, "I'm not suffering! I'm not suffering!"

With this joke, I do not mean that utilitarianism is a joke or that utilitarians go around putting animals and people out of their misery. Rather, something about the attitude of the biker reminds me of the fundamental attitude of utilitarianism; that is, humans and animals are disposable. Their true value does not consist in who they are. As I mentioned earlier, this is the egalitarian aspect that renders utilitarianism so attractive. However, there is a price to pay for that egalitarian attitude. Moral value for utilitarians is something that makes sense, or that we can speak of, in terms of the total amount of pleasure or happiness. A being is not morally valuable in itself. When functional, sentient beings are morally important because they can contribute to the promotion of aggregate utility, but when they're "broken," their moral value diminishes and often is even lost. This consideration is very peculiar, to put it candidly. But it is true that for utilitarians sentient beings are not special in their own right. Individuals are not valuable *qua* individuals. What really counts, in the case of preference utilitarianism, is satisfaction of the preferences of the greatest number of beings that have preferences, the aggregate satisfaction of preference. What this means is that, as in the joke, following utilitarian ethics, given certain circumstances, we would have an obligation to kill a person or a fetus or an infant or an animal if the greatest good for the greatest number is thereby promoted. As long as the preference of the greatest number is satisfied, anything is in principle permissible. In the biker joke, the biker is committed to a moral view that the life of a moribund being is futile when continuing his existence will bring more unhappiness than happiness. And so a bullet will take care of it. His friendship with his companion dog becomes, in a sense, insignificant. As Tom Regan pointed out, "For the utilitarian, you and I . . . have no value as individuals and thus no equal value. What has value is what goes into us, what we serve as receptacle for: our feelings of satisfaction have positive value, our feelings of frustration negative value."[17] To be sure, this kind of criticism is not novel, but it is still a telling criticism.

Consider also an example from Bernard Williams's "A Critique of Utilitarianism."[18] Williams argues that since its main concern is whether or not the consequences of our actions lead to the greatest good for the greatest number, utilitarianism argues that the motive of our actions is unimportant. Thus, there is no distinction between a person doing an act because she freely wants to do it, a person forcing another to do an act, and a person accidentally doing an act. From a utilitarian point of view, there shouldn't be a distinction because the main concern is whether or not the consequences of a person's action promote aggregate utility. To put it another way, it is not important whether a person wants to act in a certain way on purpose or under compulsion to perform that action. All that matters are the consequences of his actions. Williams thinks that one of the problems with utilitarianism is that it makes us discount our moral feelings. Consider Jim, a man confronted by the following predicament. Jim is forced to decide between killing one person to save the lives of ten people or not killing that person, in which case ten people will be killed. Utilitarianism argues that Jim has a clear moral obligation to kill one and save the rest because in so doing he will maximize utility. Now of course situations are seldom that straightforward in real life. But assuming it is a straightforward matter—kill one to save ten or else ten will die—utilitarians will naturally say that Jim has a moral obligation to kill one person to save ten people. Again, assuming that it is crystal clear that killing one person will lead to the greatest good for the greatest number, utilitarians argue that the point in morality is precisely to maximize utility, and that's the end of the story. If Jim, for example, feels badly about killing one person, according to utilitarianism, he should discount this feeling as irrelevant. But, as Williams points out, Jim (or the biker or you or I) should not discount feelings because it is of the utmost importance to give weight to moral feelings, especially in Jim's situation, where he will simply not be able to live with himself for having killed a person. Now the serious problem with utilitarianism is that if Jim decides to do the "lesser evil" and kill one person, he will, after all, have *killed* a person. If he refuses, he can at least do all he can to save the other ten. Even if he fails, *he* won't have killed anyone. But this is at odds with utilitarianism, which argues that the lesser evil, killing a person, is the right moral decision. Consequently, it is in this sense that utilitarians undermine the role of moral feelings. Accordingly, following our feelings often leads to undesirable consequences, as in the example just given where ten lives are lost. And I should also point out that our moral feelings are not necessarily reliable because feelings are subjective and often biased. However, I argue that moral feelings have a crucial role in moral understanding. They can help us see what is morally relevant in a given situation. Guilt makes us aware of our moral faults, and compassion and sympathy can reveal that others need our help and understanding. One obvious objection to this line of argument is this: Assume that I was brought up in a racist society; then my feelings would very likely be a reflection of that society's values. Thus, utilitarianism purports to guarantee a satisfactory outcome by evaluating moral issues on the basis of utility. This is because feelings lead us in many directions, unlike the objectivity of satisfying the preference of the greatest number.

However, my response to this objection is that it is difficult to know that we have to help others if we walk around with such ideas of duty or maximization of utility. Considering the same hypothesis that I was brought up in a racist society, my goal will be to maximize utility only for the greatest number of people like me. Thus, doing morality by way of calculation of utility is not an advantage over relying upon moral feelings. It is through our moral feelings that we become aware of others and their needs. Moral feelings can guide us to the right action. Uneasiness is good evidence that a certain decision is immoral. Empathy allows us to see what is morally important for others. We often sense that certain actions are wrong or right. And most importantly, moral feelings can help motivate us to perform the right action. Following rules that are imposed upon us is one thing; performing an action because we feel it is the right way to behave is another. The approach that I advocate here is that of morality as a system of virtuous actions. The acquisition of virtuous moral character will enable us to know which action is right because the story does not end at the maximization of utility.

Putting the foregoing discussion in perspective, utilitarianism is at the forefront of the animal rights movement. Many moral thinkers of utilitarian bent like Singer argue that our current treatment of animals is immoral and that we are morally required to be vegetarians. In a strange but coherent way, they argue this way because the maximization of aggregate preference principle demands it. At the risk of prompting the question "So, what's wrong with that?" I want to emphasize that utilitarians do not argue that we ought to become vegetarians because they love animals or they feel compassion for them. What is wrong about this approach, in my view, is its unhuman coldness. By coldness I mean this: If I love my child or my dog, for example, I treat them with respect. But why? Certainly not because I calculate their preferences. I don't give them respect because I wish to maximize overall utility. What kind of individual would I be? Perhaps Mr. Spock, the character of the popular TV series *Star Trek* played by actor Leonard Nimoy, can bring the wrongness of the utilitarian attitude to light.[19] Mr. Spock is half-human, half-Vulcan. His character is remembered for being very logical, to the point of almost being unemotional. His character dies for the first time in *Star Trek II: The Wrath of Khan*, where in the concluding scene, the Starship Enterprise has been damaged. To fix it, Spock enters the engine room, where he is exposed to lethal radiation. Before dying, he speaks to Admiral Kirk through the doors:

> McCoy: [Kirk runs in to the engine room and sees Spock inside the reactor compartment. He rushes over but McCoy and Scotty hold him back] No! You'll flood the whole compartment!
>
> Kirk: He'll die!
>
> Scotty: Sir! He's dead already.
>
> McCoy: It's too late.
>
> [They let go and Kirk walks to the glass and pushes the intercom button]
>
> Kirk: Spock!
>
> [Spock slowly walks over to the glass and pushes the intercom]
>
> Spock: The ship . . . out of danger?
>
> Kirk: Yes.
>
> Spock: Do not grieve, Admiral. It is logical. The needs of the many, outweigh . . .
>
> Kirk: The needs of the few.
>
> Spock: Or the one.
>
> Kirk: Spock.
>
> [Spock sits down]
>
> Spock: [Gasping] I have been . . . and always shall be . . . your friend.
>
> [He places a Vulcan salute on the glass]
>
> Spock: [Gasping] Live long . . . and prosper.
>
> [Spock dies]
>
> Kirk: No.[20]

Or, to go back to our biker in my joke, he is ready to kill his beloved companion dog without flinching, without having the least moral hesitancy, because what he really cares about is maximization of preference and not the intrinsic value of his dog and his relationships with him. The biker, indeed, would seem to be a utilitarian for trying to eliminate suffering. But no one really lives this way—not even the staunchest of utilitarians. At this juncture, I want to conclude by saying that in regard to our treatment of animals, utilitarian ethics leads to vegetarianism, as Peter Singer argues. We ought to be vegetarians, not for the sake of animals' well-being, but rather for the sake of maximizing aggregate utility. Utilitarianism does not recognize, for example, compassion, empathy, or other moral sentiments as useful guides to morality. I argue here that if we are serious about the suffering of animals, then utilitarianism does not help. Concerning ourselves with the suffering of animals (or people) requires caring for individuals. But it seems to me impossible to care for others if we do not care about our moral character first.

The foregoing describes the way utilitarianism works. What counts in morality is the end result of one's actions, not the motives of one's actions. In Singer's view, actions are deemed right through their capacity to further the preference of all sentient beings and wrong if they frustrate overall preferences. Consequently, as long as one's action produces a favorable balance between utility and disutility, that action is morally permissible and indeed required—even if the action involves treating someone unfairly. Moreover, Singer accuses those who participate in animal exploitation of being speciesists. Yet he is guilty of speciesism himself because for him it is acceptable to kill an animal if it is done in a "humane" way because animals do not have an interest in pursuing life like humans. Animals are merely interested in not suffering, but continuing their existence is not their concern because they have no such concept. Singer argues that animals (and infants too) are sentient beings but are neither rational nor self-conscious. He writes, "The most plausible arguments for attributing a right to life to a being apply only if there is some awareness of oneself as a being existing over time, or as a continuing mental self."[21] This is a rather odd view because according to Singer, on the one hand we should respect animals to the point of becoming vegetarians, but at the same time we could kill them and then eat them because animals lack a sense of continuing self. But this view is itself speciesist; for it implies that only those beings that have a notion of existing over time are morally important.[22]

CONCLUSION

In this chapter, I have pointed out that applying the principle of utility to the question of how we should treat non-human animals has two fundamental problems that render it unacceptable. First, it is frighteningly unemotional, like Mr. Spock—and thus it is difficult to embrace it because, unlike Mr. Spock, our moral life is of tremendous importance when we consider our moral attitude toward others. And second, in following the advice of utilitarianism, one may find oneself reluctant to carry out an action while obligated to do it. In other words, utilitarianism is doubly defective in that it is unemotional and lacks conative power. In the next chapter, I want to further question a moral symmetry proposed by utilitarians. By "moral symmetry" I refer to the notion that humans and animals deserve equal moral consideration.

NOTES

1. Peter Singer, *Animal Liberation: A New Ethics for Our Treatment of Animals* (New York: Random House, 1975); Gaverick Matheny, "Utilitarianism and Animals," in *In Defense of Animals: The Second Wave*, ed. Peter Singer (Malden, MA: Blackwell Publishing, 2002), 13–25; Gaverick Matheny, "Expected Utility, Contributory Causation, and Vegetarianism," *Journal of Applied Philosophy* 19 (2002): 293–297.
2. Jeremy Bentham, *Introduction to the Principles of Morals and Legislation* (1789; repr., New York: Dover, 2007), 1.
3. Bentham, *Introduction*, 1.
4. Peter Singer, *The Point of View of the Universe*, coauthored with Katarzyna de Lazari-Radek (Oxford: Oxford University Press, 2016).
5. See Bentham, *An Introduction*, and John Stuart Mill, *Utilitarianism*, 1st ed. (1863; repr., Hackett Publishing Company).
6. Peter Singer, *Practical Ethics*, 2nd ed. (Cambridge: Cambridge University Press, 1993), 13.
7. Singer, "Utilitarianism and Vegetarianism," *Philosophy and Public Affairs* 9 (1980), 137.
8. Another version regards pleasure as utility, and suffering or pain as disutility.
9. Singer, *Practical Ethics*, 14.
10. Peter Singer, "All Animals Are Equal," *Philosophic Exchange* 5, no. 1, article 6 (1974): 107.
11. Singer, "All Animals," 107.
12. Although utilitarians state this, they also admit that in principle, killing an animal for food is not wrong if done in ways that avoid pain.
13. Singer, "Utilitarianism and Vegetarianism," 327–328.
14. In a personal email to Singer, I asked him if that is still his view or if he changed his mind, and he replied, "No, that is still my view, although I think that in almost all circumstances it is better to avoid eating them."
15. This is also a controversial point because, in most cases, food can be shipped everywhere, and those who do not have anything at all typically do not have the means to rear animals. At any rate, I do not know of any examples where eating animals might be morally justified other than being stranded on a desert island on which plants do not grow, but for some reason animals abound.
16. See Singer, "All Animals Are Equal."
17. Tom Regan, *The Case For Animal Rights* (Berkeley: University of California Press, 2004), 109.
18. See Bernard Williams, "A Critique of Utilitarianism," in *Utilitarianism For and Against*, ed. J. J. C. Smart and Bernard Williams (Cambridge: Cambridge University Press, 1973), 77–150, especially 75.
19. There's a collection of essays on the ethics of *Star Trek* titled *Star Trek and Philosophy: The Wrath of Kant* focused on Mr. Spock's somehow utilitarian attitude.

20. *Star Trek II: The Wrath of Khan* (1982).
21. Singer, excerpted from *Practical Ethics*, 2nd edition (Cambridge: Cambridge University Press, 1993), 175–217.
22. See also Chappell, "In Defense of Speciesism," in *Human Lives: Critical Essays on Consequentialist Bioethics*, ed. David S. Odenberg and Jaqueline A. Laing (London: Macmillian, 1997), 98; and Gordon Preece, "The Unthinkable & Unbelievable Singer," in *Rethinking Peter Singer: A Christian Critique*, ed. Gordon Preece (Downers Grove, IL: InterVarsity Press, 2002).

Chapter Three

Eating People and Eating Animals

UTILITARIANS AND ANIMALS

Singer (like many others) suggests that all sentient beings should be given equal moral consideration. Long gone are the days when people would enslave other people because they happened to be part of a different race or group or discriminate against members of a different gender or sexual preference. Unfortunately, humanity has not completely eradicated all racism and discrimination. However, nowadays virtually all sensible individuals recognize the evil of racism, discrimination, and prejudice. Giving all members of the human species equal moral worth and consideration has turned out to be a good idea. Not too long ago in our history, many people believed they had a moral justification for discriminating against others on the basis of certain differences among individuals. Fortunately, we now recognize that since human beings are not all equal in many respects, it would seem unwise to ground equality in humanity. An intelligent reason to grant equal consideration was to get to the heart of what really counts. Does height or color or gender matter? No. Then what is the relevant characteristic, the lowest common moral denominator, possessed by all humans that confers upon them moral equality? The answer is to consider what makes certain acts wrong. For example, what is it that makes slavery immoral? It is immoral because individuals have preferences, and their preference is to not be enslaved. And this preference is an expression of one's capacity to live a life of enjoyment or a life of misery. Arguably, a life as a slave is a life of suffering.[1] Since no one desires to suffer, we should respect this preference. Thus, sentience is the ground for morality. And if this is right, then it would be hypocritical—in fact, it would be immoral—to deny equal consideration to animals, who are also sentient creatures. In other words, if we give importance to sentience, then everything that has sentience is morally important.

This argument, that we should give animals equal moral consideration, implies that denying equal moral consideration to those beings that are sentient is clearly a form of discrimination that some refer to as speciesism.[2] A speciesist is one who discriminates against members of species different from one's own. It is to put the interest of one's own species above all others. Just like a white supremacist discriminates against members of other races, a speciesist discriminates against other species. In this context, a human being who exploits or eats animals is a speciesist, for it is his assumption that the human species is superior to all others so that it is morally permissible to eat or exploit members of any non-human animal species. Certainly, in my view it is an admirable aspect of utilitarianism to point out that many commit this moral error known as speciesism.

When we come to recognize this moral error, perhaps even logical error, we should want to correct it. The way to correct it is to apply consistently the principle of equal moral consideration for all members of the human race to the way we treat other species. The result is that we condemn racism because although the parties involved might have external differences, such as skin color, height, intelligence, and so on, they all are capable of suffering. Causing gratuitous suffering is immoral. Racism causes people to suffer. Consequently, racism is immoral. And by the same token, since animals are sentient beings (at least most animals that people typically eat), to be morally consistent, it is immoral to cause them gratuitous suffering. Therefore, we have a moral obligation to become vegetarians. Many utilitarians like Peter Singer also argue on the same principle that we have an obligation to avoid using animals for scientific experiments, clothing, and other purposes that might involve animal suffering.

EATING ANIMALS AND PEOPLE

Utilitarians argue that all suffering, whether experienced by human or non-human animals, is equally bad, irrespective of the sufferer. This implies a moral symmetry between animals and humans; if we give all humans moral consideration on the basis of the fact that they all are sentient, then we must also respect animals for the same reason. In questioning this moral symmetry, I want to refer to an article by Cora Diamond, "Eating Meat and Eating People," where Diamond refers to the argument in favor of vegetarianism used by many utilitarians as the "Singer-Regan" approach, an approach she wants to reject. (I will henceforth call it "the argument.") The thrust of Diamond's rejection is that the argument contains "fundamental confusion about moral relations between people-and-people and between people-and-animals."[3] She states that the analogy used in these types of arguments is not clear at all, and thus it is difficult to see how they move from considerations about human preferences to considerations about animal preferences. Moreover, the Singer-Regan types of arguments obscure what is really important in our relations with other people and with animals. What's fundamentally wrong about this kind of argument is that it begins by asking the wrong question: What grounds do we have to claim that humans have certain rights or a certain moral consideration while animals do not? It asks why we don't kill people or inflict suffering on them while we are willing to do just that to animals. Diamond argues, "This is a totally wrong way of beginning the discussion, because it ignores certain quite central facts—facts which, if attended to, would make it clear that rights are not what is crucial."[4]

As Diamond points out, the reason that we do not eat people is not the same reason given by the argument. It is true that people have preferences by virtue of being sentient, and they prefer not to be eaten. However, we just don't eat people simply because we do not regard them as food. And even if people wouldn't mind being food, or if they died peacefully, or if human flesh were delicious and nutritious, we would still not eat them—full stop. Except for moral philosophers of the utilitarian inclination, people refuse to eat other people due to reasons that go beyond the equal moral consideration principle proposed by the argument. But then it seems that the argument is uneven because it suggests that we ought not to eat or maltreat animals because they have equal moral importance. However, if the analogy holds for animals, and demands that we not eat them or experiment on them because doing so may deprive them of their right to equal consideration and cause them distress, then this principle should also hold for humans. Namely, eating people would turn out not to be permissible because it deprives humans of their right to equal consideration and causes them distress. But this is clearly not the reason that we do not eat people. Anyone who argues this way, Diamond says, "runs a risk of leaving altogether out of his discussion those fundamental features of our relationship to other human beings which are involved in our not eating them."[5]

We do not slaughter people for food or eat dead people even if no injustice were involved in the cause of their death. We do not eat amputated limbs (except in extraordinary cases) even if the meat were good and nutritious. But again, the reason is not because we respect people's morally relevant interests or because people are capable of pleasure and pain or are bearers of interests or because we want to maximize the overall utility.

Diamond is on point when she notes that meat eaters would be appalled at the idea of eating their companion animals but have no compunction about eating steak. One might think that this is because a dog or cat has some morally relevant characteristic that a cow or chicken may lack, but it seems clear to me that this is obviously false. In fact, there are people who house-

adopt lambs or pigs or chickens as companions. And once these animals are chosen to be companions, the idea of eating them would be horrendous to many. Furthermore, the complexity of this issue is also evident by the fact that in some parts of the world, restaurants routinely serve dogs as an entrée.

Concepts like "person," "friend," and "pet" are morally rich, because they encompass a number of complex sentiments, moral relations, and duties. The reason that we don't eat our friends is that we do not view friends as food, and this is also reason that we don't eat companion animals. By becoming companions, animals typically receive a name, a place on the couch, and a meal in a special bowl, and, at the end of their lives, they are mourned and often even given a burial. Thus, like a friend or a neighbor, a companion animal is not food. Consequently, not being food is not a principle that follows from the animal's having equal moral consideration, or having rights, but rather from our relationship with and feelings toward an animal. This seems to imply that animals have the potential to be considered and loved as much as other persons. We do not have the same attachment, for example, to plants or other objects that we might cherish for sentimental reasons. Animals that we come to love are like the people we love. This is certainly an aspect that the argument fails to capture.

Reflecting on the foregoing discussion, I want to add a few words about defending animal rights on utilitarian grounds. Utilitarianism has a fatal flaw that hinders, rather than helps, the cause for animals. The flaw is that it blinds us to what is morally important about our relationship with others. It asks us to care about animals' suffering, to become vegetarians, and to oppose animal exploitation; but the reason it asks us this stems from what utilitarians believe to be the fundamental aspect of morality—that is, aggregate satisfaction of preference. What follows from this principle is that, in certain circumstances, it is preferable, and thus morally permissible or even required, to kill and eat animals and use them as subjects of scientific research. The point for utilitarians, after all, is not that life is precious or sacred. Rather, the greatest good for the greatest number is, perhaps, not sacred but precious. This principle also applies to humans. According to utilitarianism, certain marginal cases are no longer considered as persons. Consequently it would not be immoral to let them die, provided that their death is justified by the greatest good for the greatest number principle. Again, for utilitarianism, life itself is not important; aggregate satisfaction is what counts. However, it is precisely because utilitarianism respects the greatest good for the greatest number, and not animals themselves, that by definition they cannot find anything wrong with killing animals for food or other purposes, assuming that those animals have had a happy life. In such a case, the act of tearing the flesh of a dead animal then becomes, so to speak, a neutral act.

In the foregoing discussion, I hope to have raised some questions about whether our relationship with others is a mere question of equal moral consideration and of promotion of utility. I argue that it is not. As I have shown, the argument that utilitarianism relies upon rests on a fallacious moral symmetry. The purported symmetry is that we should not eat animals because in so doing we deny them equal moral consideration. However, as I suggested, this would mean that we do not eat people for the same reason. Clearly the symmetry suggested by utilitarians breaks down, because we do not refrain from eating people because we give them equal moral consideration. Besides the fact that most of us would find the practice of eating human flesh repulsive, the reason we do not eat people is because we have an intricate relationship with others—a relation of respect, friendship, and other aspects that go beyond utility. Therefore, I argue that applying the principles of utilitarianism to the question of our treatment of animals produces unsatisfactory results. Utilitarianism is morally inadequate because it implies that the lives of others and our relationship with them are not important—preferences are.

In fact, utilitarians are not opposed to eating meat in principle because, by definition, utilitarianism does not advocate absolute moral rules. The idea is that eating animals is immoral because in many cases it causes loss of utility. But while it is immoral to inflict pain on animals because animals have an interest in avoiding suffering, and we should give animals equal consideration, killing an animal per se is not wrong, nor wrong because animals do not have an interest in continuing to exist. They have only the interest not to feel pain, but they lack the concept of existing in time. Such an interest, according to some thinkers, would require a level of rationality inherent to man. Consequently, if I raised a cow and made sure she had a great, happy life, according to utilitarianism, I would do nothing wrong if I killed and ate her, provided that I killed the cow painlessly.

Now this, in my view, is an alarming moral attitude for the following reason. It seems to me quite a bizarre notion that one could take good care of an animal to the degree that will give the animal a happy life, and then after caring for it, kill and eat it. Suppose I take good care of a cow. I would groom her, feed her good food, make sure she is healthy, and make sure she is loved and free to graze outside. How could I then kill this cow, eat her, and pretend that I cared for her? When we welcome animals in our lives, we become attached to them and we no longer view them as food. And my point is precisely that if I take good care of a being, whether human or animal, by definition I do not harm her, I do not kill her, and I do not eat her—that is what *taking care* of a being means. It is for this reason that I believe it is impossible to treat an animal well and at the same time eat it. Terms such as "ethically raised" or "humanely raised" meat are offensive misnomers. The view that an animal could be killed humanely smacks of speciesism. For it is the assumption that animals, a different species from ours, can be killed in certain circumstances because they lack a capacity that we possess, the capacity to be self-aware that we want to continue our existence. However, to reflect again on Diamond's point, if the argument were consistent, it would have to say that the reason we do not eat orphan human infants or even adults who had a pleasant life and died in an unfortunate accident is just squeamishness. But if it is not squeamishness that prevents us from eating people, but rather the recognition that humans are more than mere utility, then the argument is asymmetric.

Furthermore, according to utilitarian ethics, humans and animals are not special in their own right; they are comparable to empty containers[6] that acquire value by the amount of happiness they contain. Utilitarianism is infamous for this very principle. Since what's morally important is not the container (humans or animals) but rather overall happiness, then no act is intrinsically wrong. If an act leads to consequences that promote the greatest good for the greatest number, then that is what counts. Utilitarianism has a vision of humanity and animality as mere empty containers that can be filled with pleasure/happiness or preferences. It is a moral outlook that discounts love, compassion, and the importance of relationships. This is, in my view and in the view of many others, what is fundamentally wrong with utilitarianism and the reason for its impracticality. Historically, utilitarians have been at the forefront of the animal rights movement. However, the appearance is deceiving because it might suggest an image of utilitarians lovingly hugging puppies; but in reality, they do not care about animals that way. Rather, they care about the promotion of utility. In fact, Singer argues that infanticide can be morally permissible and there is nothing immoral about bestiality (engaging in sexual intercourse with animals). The sordid aspect of such a view is expressed by Debra Saunders: "You could say Singer's take on animal rights is: you can have sex with them, but don't eat them."[7]

Utilitarianism has an uncomfortable coldness to it—it suggests that when we do morality we should not worry about our feelings toward others or our relationship with them. Rather, we should worry about the greatest good for the greatest number. At the risk of making too bold a statement, I want to say that the principles of utilitarianism have not convinced many people except for utilitarians themselves. Consequently, utilitarianism is inadequate as a moral theory, and its acceptance does not clearly lead to the conclusion that we ought to be vegetarians.

MARGINAL CASES

Another way to think about why utilitarianism fails to be an adequate moral theory, especially when applied to our treatment of animals, is by considering the issue of marginal cases, human beings with lower-than-normal mental capacities, such as infants, fetuses, the senile, and people with cognitive disabilities. Marginal cases remind us of how close humans are to non-human animals, especially when some of our cognitive functions are diminished. Utilitarians like to point out that if we give moral consideration to human infants, the senile, the comatose, and the cognitively disabled, then we must give equal consideration to animals, since there is no known morally relevant ability that those marginal-case humans have that animals lack. For example, the typical argument regarding why it is acceptable to kill a cow for food claims that cows have no concept of self or that they are inferior in intelligence to humans; therefore, it is not wrong to kill a cow. However, infant humans also lack a concept of self. So if we accept the "awareness of a continuing-self" as a criterion, it would turn out that it is not wrong to kill a human infant. In fact, for any attributes, language, consciousness, intelligence, there exists some marginal human who lacks one or more of those attributes. Thus, utilitarians point out that characteristics such as intelligence, shape, and even species are irrelevant factors to determine moral consideration. The only relevant factor is the capacity to feel pleasure and pain. As Peter Singer puts it,

> The catch is that any such characteristic that is possessed by all human beings will not be possessed only by human beings. For example, all human beings, but not only human beings, are capable of feeling pain; and while only human beings are capable of solving complex mathematical problems, not all humans can do this.[8]

This is all well and good, except for the fact that the same philosophers have suggested that the severely intellectually disabled or infants have a lower degree of moral consideration than "normal" human beings, and that therefore harming them or even killing them is not as bad as harming or killing "normal" human beings. While utilitarians argue that we should give equal moral consideration to all sentient beings, by no means do they argue that all sentient beings ought to be treated equally. Neither do we treat other beings in accordance with fixed, universal moral rules, or by our sentimental attachment to those beings. According to utilitarianism, we should discount our personal feelings about others and consider utility instead. That is, our moral attitude toward them should not proceed from our feelings of respect, compassion, or love, but rather satisfy the preference of the greatest number or promote the greatest good/happiness for the greatest number. Again, I view this as a rather disconcerting aspect of utilitarianism. From a utilitarian standpoint it is morally permissible to kill the elderly if, say, they have dementia. Also, according to the principle of utility, given certain circumstances, killing newborns is morally permissible until they are old enough to have a sense of self. Utilitarianism argues that while infants have the capacity to feel pain, they lack the preference to continue their existence, due to the fact that they lack the relevant mental concept.

My argument is not that utilitarians disregard marginal cases. (There is an enormous literature that specifically addresses this issue and, in the end, different utilitarians have different things to say about marginal cases.) If this were so, then it would seem unfair to give a general criticism of utilitarianism's attitude toward marginal cases. However, my criticism applies to utilitarianism in general since all utilitarians agree that the promotion of utility is the sole important principle of morality. In my view, embracing utilitarian principles leads to a distorted view of the moral value of these cases. If we look at their lives—possibly we come into contact with them, and we see how they live and what matters to them—we can discover moral characteristics that render them morally important.

Many consequentialists and deontologists are hostile to the idea that animals and humans are intrinsically morally important. These philosophers typically argue that humans' or animals' significance, if any, is a function of certain characteristics of those beings. In many cases, said philosophers consider mental capacities or the lack thereof as the key aspect of moral consideration. Any moral considerations are determined on the basis of the mental attributes of the beings in question. Utilitarians, for instance, think that killing humans or animals is—all things considered—the right thing to do if it reduces suffering and promotes the preferences of the greatest number. The way this is justified is by arguing that some members of the human species are not persons but rather "non-person humans." Singer, for example, writes, "I propose to use 'person' in the sense of a rational and self-conscious being."[9] And so, a "non-person human" is a member of our species, based on biology and genetics, who is incapable of the same conscious activities possessed by "normal" individuals, such as thinking, feeling, hoping, experiencing pleasure and pain, etc.

What are some important implications? One is certainly that, for utilitarianism, the mentally disabled merit less moral consideration than "normal humans." With regard to animals, as mentioned earlier, they do not have an interest in continuing their existence since they lack such a concept, so in certain circumstances it is permissible to, say, kill them, eat them, or use them as subjects for scientific research. In a personal email to Peter Singer, I asked him,

> Dear Peter, I understand from your early work you said that animals have an interest in not suffering, but they do not have an interest in continuing their existence because they lack such a concept. Hence, in certain circumstances it is permissible to, say, kill them, eat them? Have you since changed your mind on this point?

His answer was, "No, that is still my view, although I think that in almost all circumstances it is better to avoid eating them."[10] In the previous section, I made the point that utilitarianism is problematic when applied to the question of animals because utilitarianism cares about preferences, not the value of beings.

It follows, then, that certain characteristics considered relevant for moral consideration, when missing or diminished, lead to diminished moral consideration. For example, for Singer, not all humans have equal value. He argues for a "more graduated view" that depends on certain aspects of cognitive capacity.[11] Thus, for example, Singer among others is known for taking the position that abortion and even infanticide are not as morally reprehensible as one might think. After all, fetuses and infants have not yet developed cognitive capacities comparable to those of adult humans, which would enable them to have a concept of what it means to be a person and have a future. Consequently, utilitarianism supports equal consideration of animals on the basis that they have cognitive capacities or lack them. As James Rachels puts it, "if we think it is wrong to treat a human in a certain way, because the human has certain characteristics, consistency requires that we also object to treating the non-human in that way." Rachels argues that the theory of evolution shows that between humans and other animals there is a gradient, and therefore marginal-case humans should be considered similar to non-human animals.[12] This is why Singer takes the interest of animals—and humans. In other words, the idea is that beings with equivalent mental capacities have equal claims to moral considerations.

But why should severely intellectually disabled beings have lesser moral consideration than regular humans? This seems a form of speciesism, which is the very thing that utilitarianism condemns. Edward Johnson, discussing the value of the life of animals, pointed out that many moral philosophers, starting from Mill, have argued that the lives of animals are less important than human life. Mill famously declared that it "is better to be a human being dissatisfied than a pig satisfied."[13] As Johnson put it, and I concur, "How does Mill know that?"[14] I believe that John Stuart Mill was an individual of superior intelligence. Nevertheless, how could he possibly know that? If Mill were a satisfied pig, would he still think that? The view that I hold is that there is plenty special about being human or animal. All animals and humans have moral worth. Many philosophers are hostile to this idea. As an illustration, R. G. Frey writes,

> I do not regard all human life as of equal value; I do not accept that a very severely mentally-enfeebled human or an elderly human fully in the grip of senile dementia or an infant born with only half a brain has a life whose value is equal to that of a normal, adult human.[15]

And once again, how does Frey know that? Obviously, Frey here makes an arbitrary statement. The error that leads to such views is to look at sentient beings as objects of mere theoretical speculations. In other words, these views regard humans and animals as mere objects, dispensing with important moral aspects such as "sympathy, empathy, and compassion as relevant ethical and epistemological sources for human treatment of [humans and] nonhuman animals."[16] This attitude advocates that all sentient beings deserve moral consideration; but at the same time it argues that some individuals—for example, marginal cases and animals—can be treated in ways that many might regard as cruel. One implication is that, as discussed earlier, according to utilitarianism, animals do not have an interest in continuing to exist because they lack such a conception. Consequently, it would not be immoral to kill an animal in certain situations. This moral outlook is wrong. The mistake is to apply a graduated moral scale based on the mental capacities of beings. The error is to use "normal" as a baseline to assign the appropriate degree of consideration. There is no good reason to do so. The right move is to consider each type of being and see what is important from the point of view of that being and not compare it to the life of other beings. This attitude will reveal to us that it is not so clear that it is better to be Socrates dissatisfied than to be a pig satisfied.

I propose that to look at humans and animals as intrinsically morally valuable is to look more closely at animals and humans. While for utilitarians what is important is a consideration of the similarities between humans and animals—that is, the capacity to feel pain and pleasure or the fact that animals, like humans, are "subject-of-a-life"[17]—my suggestion is that we consider the differences, in the sense that the value of a being should be determined on the basis of that being's characteristics and what is important in its existence. As Richard Taylor writes, "Even the glow worms…whose cycles of existence over the millions of years seem so pointless when looked at by us, will seem utterly different to us if we can somehow try to view their existence from within."[18] I believe that the virtue of this approach—viewing one's existence from within—is that it enables us to avoid the error of using arbitrary rankings from "non-person" humans to "full-fledged" humans that some make—which is an error generated by an unjustifiable emphasis on looking at humans and animals as mere objects that can promote or suppress utility. It seems to me that this is the mistake of utilitarianism—that is, that based on their cognitive capacities, it is possible to determine the moral worth of individuals. This prompts the higher-level question, "Why should cognitive capacities decide the moral worth of an individual?" And the answer in favor of the importance of cognitive capacities must be given by an individual who possesses them and therefore believes them to be the decisive factor of moral consideration, which begs the question.

One thing that can be said (perhaps hoped) about consequentialists, and like-minded moral philosophers, is that they don't truly believe their own conclusions. Again, they assert that killing human infants is never equivalent to killing persons. Killing a child, in this view, is only wrong inasmuch as it hinders the wishes of its parents. Also not morally wrong is euthanizing victims of dementia or Alzheimer's if their care requires resources that can be used for more worthy purposes that promote aggregate preference. Peter Singer has stated that infants are sentient beings who are neither rational nor self-conscious, and therefore do not count as persons and may be killed.[19] As I mentioned earlier, a moral view that permits—in fact, a moral view that requires—killing individuals with diminished mental capacities, such as infants and adults suffering from severe mental deterioration, is the result of treating humans and animals as mere objects of theoretical speculation.

The approach that utilitarians take toward morality is procedural. Their focus is the maximization of utility. It is the utility that is important, not the individuals. This stance relies upon two points: one is that moral intuition should play no role in ethical reflection.[20] The second is that there is no ultimate meaning to the universe and to human life.[21] To the first contention, I want to say that while moral intuition sometimes obscures ethical problems, we should not be in such haste as to discount intuition altogether. Our feelings of indignation aroused by discrimination and injustice and our sympathy for less fortunate people, for example, cannot be dismissed so easily. It is because of such intuitions that we recognize (and fight) discrimination and injustice; and we help others in need. And the denial of an ultimate meaning of the universe and human life can only be speculation. Utilitarianism itself relies (perhaps tacitly) upon such intuition that we humans create meaning and that the maximization of utility ought to be recognized as a universal principle.

To see the implications of ethical theory, I want to discuss a real case. Ethics is not about theoretical speculation. It is about real problems and the ways people behave and relate with one another. The most telling case of this wrong attitude of utilitarianism can be seen in the unfortunate events in the life of Singer. After all, there is nothing more significant than observing how an ethical theory is put into practice. In this case, for all his commitment to utilitarian morality, Singer himself could not euthanize his mother, Cora Singer. Contrary to his credo, when Peter Singer's mother became ill with Alzheimer's, he opted to keep her alive. As a utilitarian, keeping alive a person who suffers from Alzheimer's is a practical question, a question of whether it is the best decision. And the best decision is one that will lead to the greatest good for the greatest number. For example, if it is clear that the resources that are required to take care of such a person will increase the happiness and diminish the suffering of many others, then as horrible as the prospect of letting one die might be, utilitarianism requires that resources be used to increase the happiness of others—which means not using those resources to keep an ill individual alive. In a 1999 profile by Michael Specter featured in the *New Yorker*, Singer makes it very clear what he thinks about humanity: "The notion that human life is sacred just because it's human life is medieval." And regarding the hopelessly ill, he adds: "The person that used to be there is gone. It doesn't matter how sad it makes us. All I am saying is that it's time to stop pretending that the world is not the way we know it to be."[22] Singer argues that the idea that human life is sacred is obsolete. These statements really encapsulate utilitarian ethics. Most people think that there is something really special about humanity; but according to utilitarianism, these people only delude themselves. For Singer, and most utilitarians, we should abandon such an idea. And the sooner we abandon it, the better we will live. By saying that we should "stop pretending that the world is not the way we know it to be," he means that we should accept that individuals are not intrinsically valuable but rather are replaceable. I argue that this is a mistake. Furthermore, I argue that it is impossible to live the way Singer suggests. As Gordon Preece points out, "Singer's rarefied rationalism of almost total impartiality is thus impossible to live out and fails his basic test of the practicality of ethics."[23] It seems to me that to "stop pretending that the world is not the way we know it to be" suggests suppressing our very nature. Mary Midgely makes a similar point:

> Feeling is an essential part of our moral life, though of course not the whole of it. Heart and mind are not enemies or alternative tools. They are complementary aspects of a single process. Whenever we seriously judge something to be wrong, strong feeling necessarily accompanies the judgment. Someone who does not have such feelings—someone who has merely a theoretical interest in morals, who doesn't feel any indignation or disgust and outrage about things like slavery and torture—has missed the point of morals altogether.[24]

But Singer is not without emotion like Mr. Spock; he just tries to deny and suppress emotion. In fact, he recognized something special in human life when he was personally touched by a family tragedy. In his interview, Michael Specter writes,

> But when Singer's mother became too ill to live alone, Singer and his sister hired a team of home health-care aides to look after her. Singer's mother has lost her ability to reason, to be a person, as he defines the term. So I asked him how a man who has written that we ought to do what is morally right without regard to proximity or family relationships could possibly spend tens of thousands of dollars a year for private care for his mother. He replied that it was "probably not the best use you could make of my money. That is true. But it does provide employment for a number of people who find something worthwhile in what they're doing."[25]

I do not intend this discussion as a criticism of Singer's "moral inversion" just to score "academic points." Rather, my intention is to bring into view an important aspect of morality that utilitarianism discounts: that highly rational and impersonal theories do not help us understand the moral worth of humans and animals. The moral outlook proposed by utilitarianism, in fact, hides the aspects that are of most importance in morality, and this is exemplified by Singer's personal life. Singer's response to this situation was not controlled by the rational, preference-calculating utilitarian philosopher, but rather by an individual—a son—who understood the moral worth of human beings, which he expressed by an act of love. But in terms of his own doctrine, Singer broke the rules. Singer's mother became so ill that she no longer recognized her children or friends. She lost the ability to reason. In such a state, according to Singer's view, she was no longer a person. The money and attention it took to care for her could have been spent to lower the suffering of many other beings, in accordance with the principles of utilitarianism. However, Singer and his sister decided instead to hire a home healthcare team to look after their mother, spending significant amounts of money—as good children are supposed to do, I may add. As I said, I am not mentioning this because I regard Singer's actions as hypocritical. On the contrary, I believe that Singer came to realize, by way of unfortunate personal circumstances, that human beings do not come in higher or lower moral categories based on their cognitive capacities, but that they all have equal moral standing. I find it rather fascinating that in this difficult life event, Singer seemed to shift from the preference-calculating, rational philosopher to a virtuous moral philosopher who would make Aristotle proud. He seemed to abandon the idea that what counts about individuals is the satisfaction of their preferences and recognized that individuals are special in their own right. In other words, with his actions, he reversed what he proposed in his published work because his actions were guided by love, compassion, empathy, and other moral sentiments and virtues.

Although many have questioned inconsistencies between Singer's actions and his theory, Singer has always responded in ways consistent with his theory. In Specter's piece on him in *The New Yorker*, Specter quotes Singer as saying, "I think this has made me see how the issues of someone with these kinds of problems are really very difficult... Perhaps it is more difficult than I thought before, because it is different when it's your mother."[26] Indeed, the difference as I argue is that theories often make you morally blind, while our direct relationship with others (humans as well as animals) reveals the true worth of individuals. When the individual in question is your mother or another who is close to you, utilitarian calculations break down. As Alice Crary argues, "A concept of what is humanly important is the right reference point for understanding the expressiveness of all human beings, without regard to how well or poorly endowed they are mentally."[27] That is to say, people and animals are more than mere empty containers that we fill with preferences/pleasure/happiness. By paying attention to others and recognizing what is significant in their lives, we realize the true source of the worth of persons: their inner preciousness and uniqueness. It is precisely a glimpse of the uniqueness of humans and animals that reveals to us "what matters in their lives" rests upon the kind of creatures they are. Once this glimpse is achieved, we see with clarity that humanity and animality are important regardless of mental capacities or other characteristics.

When we come to realize the importance of being humans and being animals by considering, as important individuals, what they need and what is important in their lives, rather than regarding them as mere objects of philosophical speculation, we will come to see that we are not justified in killing them or maltreating them even if they are marginal cases or animals. This is what makes people care and love for their companion animals, their clear vision that animals are morally important despite lacking sophisticated mental endowments. This event, I believe, illustrates the wrongness of Mill's statement that it is better to be Socrates unsatisfied than a pig satisfied. It's very important to emphasize again that the love you have for a person or an animal is one reason why you would never kill her, and the reason you love them is the inner worth of the humans and animals. When you love someone, you are enabled by love to clearly see his inner worth. Moreover, you come to realize that the person or animal has this inner worth whether or not you love him. Utilitarianism misses this point. The calculations that utilitarianism makes do not apply in real life. It is interesting that at the end of his article, Michael Specter brings into the conversation Bernard Williams, whose views of utilitarianism I discussed earlier. Williams says,

> You can't make these calculations and comparisons in real life. It's bluff, Williams told me [told Michael Specter]. One of the reasons [Singer's] approach is so popular is that it reduces all moral puzzlement to a formula. You remove puzzlement and doubt and conflict of values, and it's in the scientific spirit. People seem to think it will all add up, but it never does, because humans never do.[28]

The last words of this quote—"because humans never do"—are crucial. That is to say, morality conceived as a formula fails because abstract reasoning cannot capture the moral complexity of humanity. Singer's unfortunate life events exemplify this. He showed us that moral puzzlements require more than formulas; they require attentiveness, love, care, and a conception of human beings as intrinsically valuable. Sadly, Singer's disappointing response to this discrepancy between his actions and his philosophy is that it doesn't mean that his doctrine is wrong; it only means that Peter Singer disobeyed the rules of utilitarianism in the case of his mother and acted unethically. Here are his words:

> Suppose, however, that it were crystal clear that the money could do more good elsewhere. Then I would be doing wrong in spending it on my mother,

just as I do wrong when I spend, on myself or my family, money that could do more good if donated to an organization that helps people in much greater need than we are. I freely admit to not doing all that I should; but I could do it, and the fact that I do not do it does not vitiate the claim that it is what I should do.[29]

This answer is frustrating and shows precisely why utilitarianism fails to be a reliable moral guidance. For example, in the event that our wives, children, or friends become ill, and thus become non-persons, will the utilitarian do what he believes to be the morally right thing and allow them to die? This is precisely what utilitarianism has to offer.

CONCLUSION

In this chapter, I discussed a real-life application of utilitarianism; and as we have seen, the principle of utility has serious shortcomings. If Singer's personal experience does not negate his theory, how many such actions would it take to negate it? If Singer is convinced that he wronged the greater good when he decided to care for his mother, does he also think that he has experienced moral guilt by caring for her? At any rate, in *Practical Ethics*, Singer writes that "ethics is not an ideal system that is noble in theory but no good in practice. The reverse is closer to the truth: an ethical judgment that is no good in practice must suffer from a theoretical defect."[30] It would seem that by his own definition his action toward his mother negates his ethical theory. Singer's critics are looking for an explanation of his moral discrepancy. The explanation is that Singer did not euthanize his mother because he loves her, and love made him see that his moral theory is incapable of capturing the importance of being human. It is clear, then, that if utilitarians are sincere in their desire to bring about the greatest good for the greatest number of sentient beings, they must abandon their view that the mere fact of being human or animal is not morally important. Thus, as I have argued, utilitarianism is not a viable ethical theory that can make sense of the question of our treatment of animals because it is not interested in our love for, and relationship with, animals and people, but rather in satisfying preferences or happiness for the greatest number.

NOTES

1. Some might object to this statement by saying that not all slavery causes suffering. They might point out that in some cases slaves were treated decently, were given shelter, food, etc., and therefore being a slave in some cases would not be the worst evil in the world. But here I am referring to slavery in the worst connotation of the term. I am therefore not referring to earning a salary as a servant, but rather to being forced to serve others against one's will.

2. The term "speciesism" was first introduced by Richard Ryder in the 1970s. Singer adopted and popularized it. Ryder, Singer, and others have claimed that speciesism is like racism, sexism, and other forms of discrimination and prejudice.

3. Cora Diamond, "Eating Meat and Eating People," *Philosophy* 53, no. 206 (1978): 466. In the original quote, "people and people and people and animals" do not appear hyphenated. I added the hyphens to make the comparison clearer for the reader.

4. Ibid., 467.

5. Ibid., 467.

6. This is an analogy used by Tom Regan.

7. Debra Saunders, "One Man's Animal Husbandry," SFGATE, March 20, 2001, https://www.sfgate.com/opinion/saunders/article/One-Man-s-Animal-Husbandry-3316192.php.

8. Singer, *All Animals Are Equal,* 111.

9. Singer, *Practical Ethics*, 87.

10. Personal e-mail to Peter Singer, March 29, 2016.

11. See Eva Feder Kittay and Licia Carlson, eds., *Cognitive Disability and Its Challenge to Moral Philosophy* (Hoboken, NJ: Wiley-Blackwell, 2010), 331–334.

12. James Rachels, *Created from Animals: The Moral Implications of Darwinism* (Oxford: Oxford University Press, 1991).

13. Mill, *Utilitarianism*, 65.

14. Edward Johnson, "Life, Death, and Animals," in *Ethics and Animals: Contemporary Issues in Biomedicine, Ethics, and Society* ed. H. B. Miller and W. H. Williams (New York: Humana Press, 1983), 123.

15. R. G. Frey, "The Case against Animal Rights," in *Animal Rights and Human Obligations*, ed. Tom Regan and Peter Singer (Upper Saddle River, NJ: Prentice-Hall, 1989), 116.

16. Josephine Donovan, "Feminism and the Treatment of Animals: From Care to Dialogue," *Signs* 31, no. 2 (Winter 2006): 306.

17. See Tom Regan's *The Case for Animal Rights* (Berkeley: University of California Press, 1983).

18. Richard Taylor, *Good and Evil* (Amherst, NY: Prometheus Books, 1999).

19. See, for example, Singer, *Practical Ethics*, 170–174 and 183–184.

20. Both Hare and Singer reject the importance of moral intuition and argue that they should be rejected if they conflict with the utilitarian calculus: Richard Hare, *Moral Thinking* (Oxford: Oxford University Press, 1982), 166; and Singer and Kuhse, "More on Euthanasia," 172–173.

21. Singer, *Practical Ethics*, 331.

22. Michael Specter, "The Dangerous Philosopher," *The New Yorker* (September 6, 1999), https://www.newyorker.com/magazine/1999/09/06/the-dangerous-philosopher.

23. Gordon Preece, *Rethinking Peter Singer*, 23.

24. Mary Midgley, "Biotechnology and Monstrosity," 9.

25. Specter, "The Dangerous Philosopher," 55

26. Ibid., 55.

27. Alice Crary, *Inside Ethics: On the Demands of Moral Thought* (Cambridge: Harvard University Press, 2016), 144–145.

28. Ibid., 55.

29. Deen Chatterjee, *The Ethics of Assistance* (Cambridge: Cambridge University Press, 2004), 29.

30. Singer, *Practical Ethics*, 2.

Chapter Four

A New Horizon

Virtue Ethics

In the last two chapters, I tried to show respectively that deontology and utilitarianism are inadequate and impracticable moral theories. Consequently, they lack the resources to construct an animal-protective ethics. My critique of utilitarianism and deontology is not meant to suggest that those are the only arguments available. Rather, I wish to point out that it is those two major theories that have shaped, and continue to dominate, the animal ethics discourse. It is my view here that in order to construct a viable animal ethics it is necessary to move beyond those theories. But what I mean specifically is moving beyond their erroneous ways of conceiving the moral importance of individuals.

Having considered consequentialism and deontology, then, what have I got to offer? As I argued, the issue with deontological and consequentialist approaches is that in order to be impartial, their procedures are very impersonal, and consequently leave out of their theorizing many important factors that we need in morality. Understanding moral life and the life of animals requires a richer approach than absolute rules or calculating the amount of happiness or preference. When we theorize, we don't notice the nuances of interacting with others and what is morally appropriate. If we are told that in considering our relationship with others we should focus on the maximization of utility or that we must strictly follow universal rules, we will never be able to overcome our bias toward animals. The bias is embedded in the very moral views I criticize here. Those views distract our attention from individuals and instead focus on rights, rules, and obligations. Obviously I am not arguing that rights, rules, and obligations are unimportant. I only suggest that a successful animal ethics should be based on a wider approach that includes the importance of relationships, the concept of good, and our moral character. As an example, when a person or an animal suffers and is in need of my help, what motivates me to act is certainly not a consideration of the way my action might maximize utility or minimize disutility or the realization that I might have an objective duty to help. These considerations do not guarantee that I do help. Rather, I am motivated by my being compassionate, empathetic, and just, and by the appreciation that such a person or animal is important in his or her own right.

Therefore, I gesture in the direction of a virtue-oriented approach. As I see it, a virtue-oriented approach ideally encompasses principles familiar to such moral views as care ethics, feminist ethics, and virtue ethics—views that do not conform to the rationalistic moral theories derived from Kant, and Bentham—in other words, theories that I refer to as non-aretaic. My virtue-based approach is the idea that morality must begin by conceptions of cooperation, the good, and what a good individual is, as opposed to duty, rights, and utility. The salient difference—and the crucial difference—between these two moral outlooks is that non-aretaic theories can only tell us what to do based on their respective, self-contained theories; they give us prescriptions that we may accept or be reluctant to follow because they are merely external principles.

The point of this book is to set a case for ethical veganism arguing that proper conception of morality leads to the conclusion that in most cases it is wrong not to be a vegan. My general approach is a virtue-based ethics; this approach has an advantage over other moral theories, because it focuses on moral practice and education. By practicing good moral behavior, we acquire important moral virtues and become internally moved to be good and act appropriately. As I will show, virtue ethics is the correct approach to morality. By showing the necessity of having the virtues, particularly those of compassion, care, temperance, and magnanimity, one becomes sensitive to unnecessary cruelty and suffering and will embrace ethical veganism. The practices of eating animals and using them in various aspects of our lives typically stem from vices such as cruelty, injustice, lack of compassion, lack of temperance, and lack of empathy. When I say "typically" here I mean that eating animals and their by-products is a wrong practice for those who have readily available access to plant food. I am not suggesting, for example, that it is immoral to eat animals and their by-products if there is nothing else around to eat. The only scenario that comes to mind is that of being stranded on a desert island and forced to eat animals to survive. But in that case, it would seem odd that animals exist in an environment where plants don't grow at all. Note, however, that even assuming there is no other food around, it does not follow that eating animals is right. Perhaps it would be necessary, but being right is an entirely different question. At any rate, I will further explore this issue later. My argument here is that (except in extreme cases) eating meat and using animal by-products is a morally bankrupt practice. In short, it is wrong not to be a vegan.

ON MORALITY AND THE DISCIPLINE OF NON-ARETAIC AUTHORITIES

Some people do not care about morality unless they are affected directly. Other people want to be told precisely how to act. Consequentialism and deontology represent two examples of moral authorities that have shaped much of our moral thinking. Supposedly, they offer practical ways to make moral decisions. Some might say that such theories offer reliable directions to make moral decisions. Resolving moral problems is hard, so a theory that can precisely guide us to the right moral direction, like a moral GPS, is certainly a prevalent theory. Reliability, among many other aspects, is an alleged feature of consequentialism and deontology. An alternative approach to morality is virtue ethics (VE), which was cast aside and marginalized by modern moral philosophy[1] for a long time. The factors that led to the marginalization of VE are many and complex. Some suggest that VE had a difficult relationship with early Christian philosophers and later on with early modern philosophers. Also, some have argued that VE was abandoned because of a transition away from Aristotelian philosophy, or because it was found to have theoretical problems. Especially in the early modern period, the utilitarianism of Jeremy Bentham and the deontology of Kant overshadowed VE and led it to its decline.[2]

In my view, however, the main reason that VE was abandoned is its being misunderstood. Traditionally, VE is criticized because it does not begin with the question "Which act is the right one?" or "What does duty demand of me?" but rather with "How should I live?" or "What kind of person should I be to live a good life?" and "What is the good life?" It was thus an arbitrary decision that a proper moral theory must be focused on right action and duty. Consequently, VE was labeled as inadequate. No doubt, VE is very concerned about our moral character, though it is not limited to it. It is interesting to note that given the popularity of theories such as act or preference utilitarianism and Kantian ethics, and the criticisms waged against virtue ethics, moral philosophers seem to regard having a virtuous character as something of secondary importance. Indeed, many moral philosophers, from Kant to Singer, have denied the reliability of virtues such as compassion, temperance, or empathy as guiding forces to correct moral deliberation. Modern moral systems emphasize the importance of detached and sometimes sterile or legalistic reasoning to arrive at universal moral laws purported to direct us to make the right moral decision; or, in the case of consequentialist theories, they assure us that in morality we should only worry about the consequences of our actions and the ways they affect aggregate happiness. Kant's example of not lying to the murderer at the door and Singer's endorsement of infanticide and bestiality bring out the sinister aspect of their moral theories.

The influence of such theories has made many moral philosophers discount questions of how to grow morally, how to become a better individual—how to excel morally—and how to acquire a moral character that will lead to a good life, and consequently to right moral decisions. This is a rather worrying aspect of morality: namely, the idea that we should not concern ourselves about acquiring admirable character traits, the importance of relationships, care, compassion, and more, because procedural theories have got us covered. As I hope to have illustrated in the previous chapters, highly rational procedure in ethics often conceals important aspects of morality. Another troublesome aspect of modern morality is that it is widely accepted that performing a right action is synonymous with doing one's duty. As Hursthouse writes, "within virtue ethics, 'good action' is *not* merely a surrogate for 'right action,' nor is it simply determined by 'action of the virtuous agent.'"[3] I agree with Hursthouse that a right action is an action that deserves praise, one that will make an agent proud of doing it. This should be distinguished from what ought to be done. I mention this point specifically because, regarding our treatment of animals, I argue that what is done to animals is wrong in this sense. Even if necessary, eating animals is not an admirable action. I realize that this last statement needs to be defended. However, I will do so in the next chapter.

Many moral philosophers lament that virtue ethics is not capable of offering precise moral guidance. This is an old but still existing criticism, which I think is misguided for two reasons. First, those who advance it are prejudicial toward VE in that they presuppose one way of thinking about morality—the way consequentialism and deontology have taught them—that is, the idea that either we must act according to universal rules or the consequences of our actions must produce the greatest good for the greatest number, or the consequences of our actions must satisfy the preferences of the greatest number of sentient beings. But why believe that morality must be understood in consequentialist or deontological terms? In fact, it does not have to be so. Virtue ethics is a distinct way of looking at morality, which argues that good character precedes evaluations of right action. Second, VE has the resources to be action guiding. Rosalind Hursthouse offers a brilliant account of this, in the form of a (V) rule: "An action is right if it is what a virtuous agent would characteristically do in the circumstances."[4]

Virtue ethics is more attuned to the nature of humans. Human beings are emotionally and psychologically complex beings—a complexity that can hardly be captured by overly rational or legalistic moral theories. In chapter 2, I pointed out, as an illustration of the issue, how Singer's own preferred approach to morality put him in an uncomfortable situation. He believes that people who suffer from dementia or Alzheimer's are no longer persons and, if their deaths will reduce overall suffering, then according to the maximum utility principle, it is permissible to euthanize them. In fact, according to the principle, it might turn out to be necessary. However, his actions were contrary to his moral belief. As discussed, I believe that Singer did the right thing. And what this real case suggests is the need to abandon such moral views and to return to a moral approach such as that of VE—which is exactly what Singer embraced by caring for his mother.

Again, I mention these theories in particular because they have dominated discussions of animal rights and influenced many people's (academics and non-academics) attitude with regard to our treatment of animals. There are other views and versions of the same theories that have advanced this discussion. However, I believe that they are all ineffective insofar as, to borrow a famous expression, awakening us from our moral slumber to the realization that our behavior toward animals is immoral. I want to show that VE has the resources to defend ethical veganism—that is, the idea that it is morally wrong to use animals for food and other purposes. Consequently, I want to offer a view according to which correct understanding of VE leads us to see that ethical veganism is an expression of virtuous character, an admirable way of living. To this end, I want to start with the current state of VE.

WHAT IS VIRTUE ETHICS?

Virtue ethics is a moral approach that differs significantly from consequentialism and deontology. Surely, deontology differs significantly from consequentialism. But both theories purport to give moral guidance in the way of showing which acts are morally permissible and which acts are not. As I illustrated earlier, both of these theories offer procedures to determine the right course of action. They also offer a standard of rightness because they tell the conditions that make actions morally right. Thus, by saying that VE is a moral approach that differs from deontology and consequentialism, I mean that its primary aim is not to be a decision procedure. Arguably, this aspect of virtue ethics is what turned many thinkers away from it for a long time, though it is the very aspect that attracted many others toward it. Virtue ethics begins with a standard of good but does not claim, at least directly or by way of some sort of calculation, to guide our actions.[5] With regard to being a standard of rightness, virtue ethics does provide the condition that makes actions right; but even this aspect differs from consequentialism and deontology. While deontology argues that actions are right just if they follow absolute moral rules, and consequentialism argues that actions are right just if they maximize aggregate happiness (or the satisfaction of rational preference), virtue ethics says that a right action is an action among those available that a perfectly virtuous human being would characteristically do under the circumstances. "Virtues" refer to admirable character traits such as moderation, fairness, courage, honesty, generosity, civility, friendliness, and wittiness.[6] To give a simple example of the way it works, consider the distinction between temperance and continence as discussed by Aristotle. The difference between a continent individual and a temperate one is that the continent has an unregulated desire for something bad, but he or she resists the temptation. For example, he or she desires to smoke tobacco, drink alcoholic beverages, and eat chocolate. This person knows that those are bad things, and it would be against reason to indulge, so he resists. Conversely, a temperate individual is not pleased by acting contrary to reason. The temperate individual simply does not have those desires.[7] He or she sees that his or her actions are measured to be conducive to the ultimate happiness. Thus virtue ethics maintains that the ultimate good is happiness, and the way human beings achieve it is through a virtuous life.

Therefore, rather than a principle, the standard of rightness for virtue ethics is to exercise the virtues to live in accordance with one's nature as a human being. The virtues are reliable and intelligent human traits; they guide one's values, emotions, attitudes, and desires according to reason. A virtuous person, for example, will avoid overeating or eating any amount and type of food just for pleasure, will not take any bribe, will repay a debt, will not be party of an unjust cause, and so on. The virtuous person is a moral exemplar. In Christianity, for example, Jesus is the moral exemplar. Christians often ask, "What would Jesus do?" in order to determine the right way to live. Nowadays, there are many interpretations of virtue ethics that in their turn differ from the original formulation of the theory given by Aristotle. Obviously, the modern world is socially and politically more complex than the Greek polis. Consequently, many contemporary virtue ethicists have interpreted Aristotle's principles in ways that make sense to the present. Thus, there are several modern interpretations of VE.[8] As Rosalind Hursthouse notes, the proponents of VE nowadays "allow themselves to regard Aristotle as just plain wrong on slaves and women." We also regard other traits, such as charity, benevolence, and others, to be on the list of virtues, despite Aristotle's failure to do so.[9] In my view, although the virtuous individual, as ideal moral agent, is often mentioned in discussion about virtue ethics, the principal aspect of the theory is the virtues themselves and acting from them.

Not all virtue ethicists argue that the right action is that which the virtuous person performs. And not all virtue ethicists agree that the right action is equivalent to the moral action. As I will discuss later, one of the many criticisms of virtue ethics is that the theory argues that the right action is right because the virtuous person performs it; but the virtuous person does not perform it because it is right. This criticism tries to show that the theory has a serious problem because it seems to suggest that certain acts are not intrinsically right or wrong; rather, they are right if they are performed by the virtuous individual, wrong if they are avoided by the virtuous individual. But then, it is noted, how can we say that, for example, saving a child from being hit by a car is not itself right? It seems that it is. But then it follows that it is not right because it is the action that the virtuous person would perform. This looks and smells like the Euthyphro Dilemma for good reason. Later I will address this criticism and argue that it is, just like the very Euthyphro Dilemma, a false dilemma.

In any case, virtue ethicists do not necessarily need to adhere to the notion that right action is right only because the virtuous person performs it. Without getting too deep into the issue at this juncture, a virtue ethicist may hold that, in fact, the virtuous person performs a certain action in a given circumstance *because* it is a right action. Other virtue ethicists instead argue that the right action is always or is typically embedded in the virtues, so that being consistent to the virtues of, say, justice, courage, and temperance, leads to the right action. Rosalind Hursthouse, for example, maintains that even a completely virtuous person might find herself in a situation in which nothing that she does is right. It might be the best option, but still not the right action. A perfect example is the unfortunate situation described in *Sophie's Choice* in which a mother must choose which of her children is to be killed by the Nazis and which is to be saved. If she fails to choose, the Nazis will kill all her children. In such a case, one cannot fail to make a choice. Even a perfectly virtuous person in a similar predicament would not be able to do what is right.

THE VIRTUE APPROACH

Virtue ethics argues that it is fruitless to try to determine the right action before we ensure that we have a good and reliable moral character. It is like putting the proverbial cart before the horse. The main point of the virtue approach is human flourishing. Many concepts, such as flourishing, have preoccupied scholars, and for obvious reasons. If flourishing is intended as blossoming like a flower, I find it to be a useful analogy. Flowers, though lacking rationality, are natural entities like humans. This suggests that just like a bud that has a course of life from seed to full-blown flower, human and non-human animals also start as seeds and eventually may flourish. In nature, we see everywhere many life forms that have distinct functions. It is true that nowadays we no longer see nature and organisms as fixed in an Aristotelian sense. Rather, many propose that this is perhaps an ancient myth, as Robert Sinsheimer writes: "We should have the potential to create new genes and new qualities yet undreamed of."[10] In an article where she comments on Sinsheimer's remark, Mary Midgley points out,

> On the whole, then, today's evolutionary biology tells us that however much we might want to have a world filled with novelties and monsters, chimeras and winged horses and three-headed dogs, we can't, because in the real environment these would not be viable life forms.[11]

Fixed forms of life and what is natural for certain organisms are thorny subjects. I think Philippa Foot's *Natural Goodness* is a brilliant example of this. Foot discusses a way to interpret the idea of flourishing, drawing from Michael Thompson, by considering what she calls a "form of life." Arguably, it is a difficult task to identify the conditions and factors that promote or thwart the flourishing of an organism. But it is not impossible. "Flourishing" means that every living organism, typically, has a way of living a "good" life or a bad one in accordance with the nature of that being, given certain internal and external factors. From inanimate objects to human beings, we notice a similar process. A seed becomes a bud and then a flower. But if it is damaged, or it lacks water, sun, and soil, obviously it will not do what is its natural course. Humans are obviously more complex than seeds, but it doesn't follow that we cannot tell what it means for a human being to flourish. A typical criticism is that it is very hard, given the history and evolution of man, to determine the conditions that make humans live a good life, and that happiness, flourishing, and eudaimonia are not precise concepts. We can start by listing conditions that are evidently conducive to a better existence. For example, human beings are not meant to be slaves. This sounds like an assertion, but in fact by looking at humans there is nothing that suggests that they are supposed to be slaves or that being slaves makes their lives better. Besides freedom, humans need friendship, affection, shelter, and a certain physical and mental fitness, among many other things. It seems undeniable that certain aspects of human existence contribute to or prevent a good life. And of course, the more difficult objection is the so-called "is/ought" problem that David Hume first pointed out. It is not obvious how one can move from a descriptive statement of how things are to a prescriptive moral statement (of how it ought to be).

Obviously, to address such an issue would require my writing an entirely different book. However, I want to try to address this issue by making the following remark. In general I agree that it is not always obvious how to move from *is* to *ought*. As John McDowell has argued, the very ability that humans possess to use practical reasoning requires contemplation of various options.[12] For example, in the bestseller *Born to Run*, Christopher McDougall argues that humans are natural born runners. Assuming that this is true, it does not follow that all people must take up running. The natural fact that humans are born to run (if it is a fact, which, as a runner, I am not trying to dispute), does not give any practical or normative weight to an individual's decision to be a runner. Hume was looking for a causal link between *is* and *ought*, just like he was looking for a causal link between events in the world. And since he could not see a link, he declared that there is no rational justification to describe events in the world as causally connected. By the same token, Hume noted, there is no link between *is* and *ought*. I am not sure what sort of "link" would have satisfied Hume. However, I think he was wrong. His mistake, I believe, stems from the fact that in the *Treatise of Human Nature*, he argued that a cause must be prior to its effect. In the *Critique of Pure Reason*, Kant showed that simultaneous causation is possible, like a ball causing a hollow on a cushion.[13] Therefore, he concluded that causation is a pure intuition of our faculty of understanding. It seems to me, then, that institutions such as lying, slavery, and torture, for example, are immoral because they hurt others. As Midgley writes,

> Institutions such as torture, or slavery . . . have moral consequences that are not accidental. We can expect those moral consequences to follow, not because of a contingent causal link (like expecting that someone may be killed by a tornado) but because they are effects that anyone who acts in this way invites and is committed to accepting.[14]

With regard to nature and options, while it is true in many cases that the nature of a being does not dictate what that being ought to do, as in McDowell's example of the wolf that acquires certain intellectual capacities, nature should not be discounted altogether.[15] It is obvious that the capacity of thinking gives humans options, but it is also true that not all options are conducive to flourishing. Taking drugs, for example, destroys one's life. Therefore, whether or not one has options, it does not mean that either option is equally conducive to flourishing.

THE COMPONENTS OF VE

Virtue ethics thus emphasizes the kind of character required for a person to flourish. As mentioned, nowadays virtue ethicists tell different stories of how we should understand a theory of virtue, each of which might slightly differ from the principles described by Aristotle's *Nichomachean Ethics*. By and large, the idea of virtue ethics makes sense by looking at the moral life in terms of activity. Aristotle thought that every activity has a final cause, and that is the good at which it aims. Taking up piano lessons, getting a college degree, learning to cook, and more seem to be disparate activities; but if Aristotle was right, the goal is still the same. The immediate goods of those activities, one might point out, are to be a good piano player, to be a cook, or to be educated. But these are not the ultimate good. They are what philosophers call instrumental goods. A good that is instrumental is something desired for its consequences rather than for its own sake alone. And since there cannot be an infinite regress of extrinsic goods, there must be a highest good at which all human activity ultimately aims.[16] This ultimate end of human life is called *eudaimonia*, typically translated as happiness or as flourishing or as the good life. But what is that? It is not pleasure, wealth, or honor, since even the achievement of these may not guarantee one's happiness. The way to understand eudaimonia is by considering the notion of a final goal, purpose, and proper function. A knife's goal, purpose, and proper function is to cut properly. So in order to achieve that goal, a good knife must be sharp, hard, and made of a material that does not rust, among other characteristics. If everything in nature has a purpose or end, then humans must have one too. Eudaimonia is the final goal and is happiness. According to Aristotle, happiness in this sense of the ultimate goal of humans involves the proper function of human life, and that is an activity of the soul that expresses genuine virtue or excellence.[17] And because humans, unlike other things in nature, are rational creatures, flourishing is achieved by acquiring a harmonious character, appropriately balanced between reason and desires. Thus, true happiness can be attained only through the cultivation of the virtues.

Standard interpretations of the *Ethics* usually have Aristotle emphasize the role of habit in conduct. That is, virtues, according to Book II, chapter 4, are identified as *hexis*; hexis are habits that are conducive to the good life. Besides habit, or custom, hexis also denotes an active condition, a state that manifests itself in action. Moral virtues arguably are the most important aspect of VE. Virtues are admirable character traits, or desirable dispositions, which contribute, among other things, to social harmony. These character traits enable us to act in accordance with reason. Virtues enable us to feel appropriately and to have the right intention in a given situation. The person whose character is not virtuous may do what appears, from the outside, like the right thing to do, but his motives will leave something to be desired. For example, a person who has acquired the virtue of honesty will usually tell the truth. Telling the truth for the right reason at the right time in the right situation is what an honest individual would do, and not because one fears the negative consequences of being found out for telling a lie. Critics of virtue ethics often object that, put this way, according to virtue ethics, something is right just because it is what the virtuous individual would do, and it is wrong just because the virtuous individual would not do it. And the problem, so it is argued, is that we can never say that certain acts are inherently good or vicious independently of what the virtuous person decides.

The criticism just described is a version of the Euthyphro dilemma. It might be recalled that in the eponymous dialogue, Euthyphro argues that the pious is what the gods love.[18] Socrates points out something that generates the dilemma: namely, either the gods love certain things because such things are pious, or certain things are pious because the gods love them. In other words, either something is loved because it is already pious or it becomes pious as a result of the act of loving it. The poor Euthyphro is confused and at first accepts that the gods love the pious because it is pious. In this case, however, what is pious is independent of the gods; namely, it pious by nature or for reasons other than the decision of the gods. The other possibility is that the gods decide that an action or a person is pious, and as a result of the gods' decision that action or person becomes pious; in this case the pious is an arbitrary judgment of the gods. Consequently, the objection goes, the pious would be just the arbitrary decision of the gods. The Euthyphro dilemma parallels the criticism of virtue ethics: If things are intrinsically right or wrong, then right and wrong are independent of the virtuous individual; but if right and wrong depend on the judgment and actions of the virtuous person, then we could never say that, for example, intentionally hurting innocent people is inherently wrong. But clearly, it seems that certain acts are just wrong and others are right. This, however, seems to me to be an unfounded criticism. Rather, it seems to me to be what is known in logic as a false dilemma or false dichotomy. This type of fallacy occurs when one is obligated to choose between two options when in reality there are more than two. If I argue that you either went to Jersey City from Manhattan by boat or by car, and you did not go by car, then it follows that you went there by boat. My argument is deductively valid. However, it commits the informal false dilemma fallacy. The reason is that it is false that you have only two options—namely, either go by car or go by boat. You could swim across the Hudson River, ride a bike, walk, etc. Regarding the Euthyphro dilemma, there is at least a third option: The gods themselves are the paradigm of piety, and so pious things reflect the gods' character. With respect to virtue ethics, then, helping an elderly person cross the street, for example, is right because the virtuous person would do it. But it does not follow that helping an elderly person cross the street is a morally neutral act that becomes right just because it is what the virtuous person would do under the circumstances. It does not follow that we cannot say, independently of the decision of the virtuous person, that such an act is right. Hursthouse proposes the (V) rule: "An action is right if it is what a virtuous agent would characteristically do in the circumstances."[19] But it seems to me plausible to say that the act itself is right because it reflects the nature embodied by the virtue in action in the circumstance. Thus, the virtue ethicist, in saying that an action is right just because the virtuous person performs it, does not need to maintain that an action is either intrinsically right or that its rightness is contingent upon the virtuous person's decision. The virtue ethicist can say that certain actions are right because they are consistent with the nature of virtue. One might object that this answer is obscure; but nevertheless it is an option, making the dilemma a false one. Certainly we need to show what virtues are and why they are important.

According to Aristotle, virtuous action is an intermediate state between two opposed vices of excess and deficiency: too much and too little are always wrong.[20] For example, courage is a mean between the excess of rashness and the deficiency of cowardice; temperance is a mean between the excess of intemperance and the deficiency of insensibility; Although the analysis may be complicated or awkward in some instances, the general idea of Aristotle's ethical doctrine is clear: Avoid extremes of all sorts and seek moderation in all things. A person may engage in a seemingly virtuous action by chance or under compulsion. His action is truly virtuous only if (1) he knows that the action is virtuous, (2) he chooses to do the action for the sake of being virtuous, and (3) his action proceeds from a firm and unchangeable character. In short, an action is truly virtuous if it is something a virtuous person would do.[21]

Flourishing, or the final goal of humans, is achieved by the exercise of virtuous actions. Thus, individuals who do not acquire the virtues are defective. Several neo-Aristotelian ethicists have dispensed with this idea altogether, proposing an agent-based VE.[22] Others might say that this component need not be taken literally. Whether acorns or human beings really have a final end decided by nature is not a concept necessary to the argument of VE. The good life for a cow is empirically different from the good life of a human being. By the same token the good life for a capable human is different from the good life of a mentally impaired individual. The point is that it is not an impossibility to determine what constitutes the good life for an individual or for a cow by studying the individual or the cow. And I find it reasonable to think that a human being with Down syndrome or one with mental retardation can achieve happiness based on individual capacities and potentials. Nor does one need be wealthy to achieve happiness. Contrary to the criticism that VE appears to be elitist, it is precisely in the lives of the less fortunate that we see examples of virtuous living. One who has enough funds to barely provide food for his family but takes the trouble to feed a hungry stranger exhibits the nobleness of character that VE describes.

The very concept of the virtues, thus, is not as problematic as some philosophers make it out to be. What I find interesting about critics of virtue ethics is that, by and large, they do not deny that certain traits of one's character, such as compassion, temperance, generosity, and so on, are desirable. Rather, they typically play down the importance of such traits in a moral theory and in their reliability.

Linda Zagzebski, for example, proposes an exemplarist VE, a form of virtue ethics based on direct reference to moral exemplars. The idea is to understand what virtues are by studying and imitating certain exemplars of virtue. For Aristotle, virtues are the means between two excesses. I accept that illustration. But there are other ways to understand virtues. I define virtues as valuable moral traits we acquire through practice and observation necessary to humans to achieve happiness. Just as any discipline requires skills, so does morality. Because morality happens socially, we can compare it to any social discipline. The goal of any discipline is to become good in particular respects and contribute to a specific social area. In morality, we want to become good so that we flourish, and this requires certain skills. As a social discipline, then, we might ask which particular skills are conducive to a good social life. Aside from a lifeboat hypothetical and particular circumstances, virtually all philosophers agree that, for example, cruelty, viciousness, and malice are not moral skills that are conducive to a good life. If, as I point out, ethics happens socially, then magnanimity, compassion, justice, benevolence, and all other character traits that have a good disposition are valuable moral skills because they are consistently conducive to happiness. Yes, circumstances might require, say, a parent lying to her child by telling him that Santa will bring a gift or that grandma is in a better place now, or for a ruler to lie to his citizens because telling the truth might lead to conflict. But the motivation for lying proceeds from certain virtues that possess a good disposition that aims at the good life. For example, the parent's lying is motivated by her love for her child, knowing that telling the truth—Santa Claus is not real, kid!—may break his heart. So the virtues are good (in the sense that they are characterized by benevolent intentions) moral skills required by humans to achieve happiness, which is what the ancients might have referred to as eudaimonia.

Therefore, it is perhaps hard, but not impossible, to define virtues. At a very practical level, we do have an idea of what it means to say that one is a liar and another sincere. Also, we understand the distinction between one who lies from a noble disposition of character—for example, one who tells her aged, dying parent that he will recover—and another who lies for a malicious, malevolent, or similar purpose—one who, for example, lies to get out of trouble or with a selfish or destructive motive. When we say that one is a chronic liar, we do not use the term arbitrarily. Rather, we say that the liar's character is not virtuous or that it is ignoble. And we recognize that an individual who lives his life by always telling the truth (except when telling the truth might hurt somebody or a lie is required for a good cause) is a trustworthy individual and socially valuable. Or, in other words, he is a virtuous individual or has virtue.

Another component of VE is the concept of practical wisdom. Once again, these principles—flourishing, the virtues, and practical wisdom—have generated a vast literature. It is not my intention here to review that literature. Insofar as my project is concerned, this literature constitutes a cumulative case for VE. Although there are different virtue theories or approaches, I believe that VE, alongside feminist and care ethics, make a cumulative case for ethical veganism. My intention is to apply VE to the question of our treatment of animals and to show the steps required to move toward veganism. Practical wisdom is the idea that a virtuous agent, besides acquiring the virtues, must also acquire an intellectual skill that enables him to make the right decisions when faced with particular moral dilemmas.

Aristotle discusses practical wisdom in Book VI of the *Nicomachean Ethics*. Practical wisdom (*phronesis*) is an intellectual virtue, a virtue of practical reasoning. Aristotle distinguishes two kinds of reasoning: theoretical reason and practical reason (VI. 1). Theoretical reason investigates the unchangeable and aims at the truth. Practical reason investigates things that are subject to change and aims at making good choices. To make good choices, not only must our reasoning be correct, but we must also have the right desires (VI. 2). The person with practical wisdom deliberates well about how to live a good life (VI. 5). So practical wisdom is "a true and reasoned state of capacity to act with regard to the things that are good or bad for man" (VI. 5).

What Practical Wisdom Involves

Practical wisdom differs from other sorts of knowledge because of both its complexity and its practical nature. Aristotle claims that an agent endowed with practical wisdom has a conception of what is good or bad in relation to what leads to human flourishing and the ability to have pertinent feeling, choice, and action in a particular situation, hence the ability to deliberate well and the ability to be moved and to act on that deliberation. Essentially, practical wisdom is the ability to deliberate with a good end. Among other things, practical wisdom involves understanding what is required in a particular situation in light of what is good. Thus, one might ask how to achieve what is good in any particular situation. And since there are no rules as to how we use knowledge of the good life to specific situations, are we not lost in a circle? Or more specifically, how can VE be universalized? But given the fact that VE tells us that if we perceive the particular facts involved in a situation and then deliberate accordingly, it does not follow that ethics is subjective, because there are truths about states of affairs that are objective and discoverable. For example, it is true that if I want to determine whether, as a virtuous individual, I should get an abortion, my deliberation may change according to the particular situation.[23] Virtue ethics starts its evaluation from objective facts about my relationship with the fetus and other persons involved, their value as individuals, and the circumstances at hand. Thus, in this sense virtuous agents may make different decisions with respect to various circumstances. Nevertheless, there are objective core facts about morality. With regard to our treatment of other beings, human and nonhuman animals, it is not the case that different virtuous agents should come up with different ways of treating them. All virtuous agents respect others—this does not change from agent to agent or from one culture to another. In fact, benevolence, as Hume pointed out, is universally recognized as a valuable virtue, and killing an innocent person is universally recognized as a vice. Lying gratuitously is never good, regardless of the culture one is in. Adultery also is never permissible, regardless of the different virtuous agent.

MORE OBJECTIONS

Aristotle argues that practical wisdom requires virtue. Without good character, we cannot understand what is truly good. But this means that knowledge of the good is not within everyone's reach. But VE is not an elitist moral view. Knowledge of the good can come in degrees. If someone is deranged or a sadist, perhaps he doesn't know what is good or bad. But most people, regardless of whether or not they are intellectually gifted, will have enough understanding of the good to make moral decisions. For example, consider Italian peasants who protected Jews from the Nazis. Arguably, these were not scholars but simple folks who understood the circumstances and acted virtuously out of love to protect other fellow humans. Most importantly, people can improve their knowledge of what is good by emulating the gestures of good people and by becoming moral people.

Another objection is that the doctrine of the mean is not precise enough to be a moral guide. But this need not be an obstacle. Aristotle didn't necessarily intend the doctrine of the mean to be a precise guide. He repeatedly states that the mean is to be determined by the virtuous agent; so the agent who possesses practical wisdom judges where the mean lies. The issue here is this: If I have practical wisdom, I know what to do. But if I do not have practical wisdom, simply telling me to do what a virtuous individual would do in the circumstances doesn't seem helpful because I don't know what the virtuous person would do. This question can be answered by pointing out that just because VE does not provide a how-to manual doesn't mean that it provides no guidance at all. Other moral theories have the same dilemma. Deontologists ask, "Will I want everyone do this?" and utilitarians ask, "Which action(s) will bring about the best consequences?" VE instead asks a series of questions: "Would this action be kind/courageous/compassionate, etc.?" the advantage of VE over non-aretaic theories is that a virtuous agent sees relevant facts about a situation and is internally motivated to act in ways that are good because they are expressions of virtue.

Tragic Dilemmas

A tragic dilemma is a situation in which a person's available actions will inevitably lead to morally undesirable consequences. The typical example of a moral dilemma is exemplified by *Sophie's Choice*; Sophie is detained in a concentration camp with her two children. The Nazis tell her that she must choose which of her children will be sent to the gas chamber. If Sophie refuses to choose, the Nazis will kill both children. At the outset I want to point out that extreme cases do not constitute legitimate criticisms of any moral theory. Whether or not Sophie is a deontologist or a utilitarian, her life will inevitably be ruined. The very fact that Sophie's available options are not options she would ideally choose shows the impossibility of any theory to give correct guidance in this kind of situation. However, I think that, contrary to criticism, virtue ethics has more to say about such a moral dilemma than other theories.

Deontological ethics would emphasize that the duty that Sophie has to both the children is equal. Giving away one child or the other would seem to be equally wrong. At the same time, Sophie has the obligation to make a choice. She has a duty to save her children, and therefore it would be wrong to choose one as opposed to the other. Letting both children be killed is also wrong. So a duty-based approach seems to be incapable of guiding Sophie.

Consequentialism does not fair better either. It might suggest that Sophie give one child to the Nazis because it is the best available option; that is, considering that utilitarianism argues that the point of morality is the greatest good for the greatest number, one child sent to the gas chamber is better than two children sent to the gas chamber. But which child should Sophie pick? Should Sophie perhaps try to determine which of her children's lives is more important than the other? Which child's death will cause the lowest amount of pain? It is hard to see how this decision could be made based on utilitarian principles. Not to mention that Sophie, if she survives, will suffer tremendous psychological trauma having to live with the knowledge that she gave one of her children to the Nazis. Utilitarian ethics, therefore, is also incapable of giving any satisfactory solution.

But what about VE? What can a virtuous person do in such a predicament? In my view, VE has an advantage over other theories here because it evaluates the issue from all angles. There seem to be different options. Obviously one option is to choose one child and save the other. But for reasons already discussed, how could she choose one as opposed to the other? Certainly another option could be to offer herself to the Nazis instead of her children. But this might not be an option, and even so it would leave her children orphans in a concentration camp. But the point is that VE is not concerned about absolute duty or achieving the best result. Rather, VE is concerned about flourishing. It seems rather extravagant, to say the least, to mention flourishing here. No one will flourish in this kind of predicament—one child will be sent to the gas chamber, and Sophie's life is going to be destroyed. But a virtuous person does what is admirable. He or she acts in a way such that he or she can look back and be proud of his or her actions.

Socrates, after all, refused Crito's offer to escape from prison and decided to face his death sentence. Crito reminds us of a consequentialist with his insistent but ineffective speech to convince Socrates to flee. Socrates, however, was not concerned about consequences, but rather was concerned about his integrity, as he reminds Crito, "It seems to me that the following statement, too, which we have been over before, still remains the same as it did previously. So examine again whether or not it still holds true for you, that it's not living that should be our priority, but living well."[24]

It seems to me that a virtuous person who found herself in Sophie's predicament would refuse to act—namely, she would refuse to choose which child would be sent to the gas chamber. Granted, such a choice would result in both children being killed. However, I think it is the virtuous choice because Sophie could not live knowing that she chose one child over the other. Children (we must remind consequentialists) are not replaceable. It is not as if one dead child is better than two dead children. Her life would be destroyed whether one child were killed or two were killed. Refusing to choose, at least, would prevent her from having to live with the notion that she was responsible for the death of one of her children. As such, if her children were both killed, and she remained alive, she would be the only one who would suffer, rather than her children. And at this point, she would even have the option of taking her own life. This is not what we want to hear from a moral theory. But when a person finds herself in a tragic dilemma through no fault of her own, unfortunately there is no way out or a best solution. Therefore, the idea of virtue ethics is that the only response to a tragic dilemma is to act in a noble way. And this seems to me to be refusing to make a choice that would cause one of the children to die, in Sophie's case.

Another criticism is that virtue ethics does not offer adequate moral guidance. When we are confronted by a moral question, we would like to have a moral compass to show us the right direction to take. This is one of the reasons why deontology and utilitarianism are very appealing moral theories; they claim to offer policies for evaluating acts. Virtue ethics, it is argued, can only advise that we do what a virtuous person would do. But virtue ethics can also provide moral direction by telling us to act according to the virtues. However, what happens when these virtues conflict with one another? Suppose you witnessed your best friend's husband being unfaithful to his wife. What would a virtuous person do? Those who criticize virtue ethics point out that in such a situation one would be totally lost because virtues often conflict with one another. It seems that the virtue of honesty advises telling your friend about her unfaithful husband; but at the same time, minding one's own business seems to be what a virtuous person characteristically does.

I think the problem with this sort of criticism stems from assessing virtue ethics using the framework of other theories. That is to say, a deontologist or a utilitarian would approach this issue by trying to determine one's duty or which act would yield maximum utility. I argue that those theories cannot provide a clear solution to the adultery problem just described. And this is not the "you too" fallacy, because I argue that virtue ethics can give a satisfactory solution.

I find it hard to imagine that deontology or utilitarianism would propose that we determine our duty according to reason or according to the maximum utility principle without personally consulting the individuals involved. A virtuous person would first of all talk to the adulterer to understand his motivation and, perhaps, discreetly inquire about her best friend's marital situation. This is not a case of not minding one's own business since it involves the life of a best friend and what is right and fair; and by witnessing the adultery you are personally involved in the situation, anyway. Unlike other moral approaches, whose procedure involves abstraction and calculation, virtue ethics suggests assessing the particular situation by communicating with the parties involved. Suppose your friend knows about her husband's escapades. Telling or not telling her would not make any difference. Or, suppose your friend is in love with her husband and oblivious of his conduct, which could destroy her. In this case it seems clear that the right thing to do—and I think virtually all honorable individuals would do the same—is to tell your friend and help her through this difficulty.

Another criticism is that VE proposes that before we can ask what the right thing to do is, we ought to be or become good individuals. To say that one should aim at becoming "a good individual" apparently has generated a great deal of confusion and skepticism among moral thinkers. But in practical terms I take it to mean that most thinkers already know that a compassionate, honest, temperate, magnanimous individual is a good individual and a callous, dishonest, intemperate, small-souled individual is not. But evidently this is not enough. In *Inventing Right and Wrong*, J. L. Mackie complains that

> as guidance about what precisely one ought to do, or even by what standard one should try to decide what one ought to do, this is too circular to be very helpful. And though Aristotle's account is filled out with detailed descriptions of many of the virtues, moral as well as intellectual, the air of indeterminacy persists. We learn the names of the pairs of contrary vices that contrast with each of the virtues, but very little about where or how to draw the dividing lines, where or how to fix the mean. As Sidgwick says, he "only indicates the whereabouts of virtue."[25]

Many others echo Mackie's criticism. Robert Louden, for example, argues that while Aristotle tells us that right acts are those that are means between extremes, it is almost impossible to determine how to apply this conception in actual situations:

> Virtues are not simply dispositions to behave in specified ways, for which rules and principles can always be cited. In addition, they involve skills of perception and articulation, situation-specific "know-how," all of which are developed only through recognizing and acting on what is relevant in concrete moral contexts as they arise. These skills of moral perception and practical reason are not completely routinizable, and so cannot be transferred from agent to agent as any sort of decision procedure....Due to the very nature of the moral virtues, there is thus a very limited amount of advice on moral quandaries that one can reasonably expect from the virtue-oriented approach.[26]

Thus, he concludes that virtue-based ethics cannot be of any use in applied ethics or in casuistry. Now this criticism is very interesting if it is meant to imply that other normative theories are preferable to VE in casuistry as reliable guides. But that does not seem to be the case. Thus this criticism ends up being a different way of saying that in morality there are extremely difficult circumstances to which no one can possibly find solutions. Consequently, traditional moral approaches of non-aretaic kinds fail to resolve extremely hard moral issues. However, virtue-oriented approaches have the advantage of showing that certain actions are the best options available—but it does not follow that they are the right things to do.

Think of a case of abortion, for example. How would a deontologist make a decision? Never kill? It would seem that deontology deems abortions wrong for two main reasons: It is the duty of parents to care for their child, not abort it, and we should treat everyone as ends in themselves, not a means to an end. To the first, what if the pregnancy was caused by rape? What if allowing the pregnancy to its full course will cause the death of the mother? What if the pregnant woman is underage and the child was conceived by error? To the second, according to Kantian ethics at least, a fetus is not a rational being; consequently, the pregnant woman does not have direct duty toward the fetus. Therefore, what should a deontologist do about abortion? Granted, contemporary deontologists might jump out of their skin upon reading this statement. They might protest that deontology has a way out of this issue. However, it seems to me that the very idea of deontology as proposing absolute moral rules does not fit well with abortion.[27] Consequentialism seems to fare a little better than deontology, but not much better. For consequentialism suggests that in considering an abortion, a woman should ponder which action (aborting or not aborting) would maximize utility or minimize disutility. This seems to me a nearly impossible task. But suppose for the sake of argument that one could come up with such a calculation. Now the fate of the fetus would depend upon some abstract calculation of an individual pregnant woman and her understanding of how aborting or not aborting will achieve maximum utility. Obviously the utilitarian would rejoin, "Yes! That's the point!" But this approach unfortunately overlooks the importance of the woman's feelings, including physical and psychological repercussions of an abortion. Surely, these aspects could be factored into a utilitarian calculation. Nevertheless, it might still turn out that the right decision is an abortion in spite of the pregnant woman's feelings about the issue. Hence, I would say that the traditional theories suffer from the problem of application, because by abstracting and focusing on rights, they overlook important aspects of a moral issue, including relationship, emotions, and more. Far from this, VE is very useful in applied ethics and casuistry. The advantage of VE over other theories, once again, is that in such cases as abortions, VE takes into consideration the particularities of specific contexts and circumstances of pregnant women. Is VE routinizable? It seems to me that it is. To say, for example, that adultery, gratuitous lying, and murder are always and under any circumstance immoral from the standpoint of VE is to say that one who possesses certain virtues—of loyalty, compassion, honesty, and temperance—does not commit such acts. There are, of course, many other examples. It seems to me to be an oft-misunderstood concept that VE is not committed to absolute rules. Not being committed to absolutes is one thing, but it does not follow that according to VE, in morality, anything goes.

A further criticism is the epistemological problem: *How do we know who is virtuous?* It is not possible to infer virtuous character simply by observing acts. Possessing virtue requires acting for the right reason *and* acting on proper desires. Surely we cannot infer character just by observing an agent's behavior. But it seems to me that the point of morality, at least insofar as this book is concerned, is not character assessment but rather virtuous action. In other words, the point of VE that I have been discussing here is that humans have a final goal in common: flourishing. As I have described it, flourishing is individual and human fulfillment. An individual should find fulfillment by choosing to live according to virtue, with good practical reasoning and sound emotions. This is the natural activity of humans.[28] Most importantly, a good human life is a social one. Consequently, VE says that flourishing is not an egotistical urge to be happy. Rather, in order to achieve it, it is necessary to treat others honestly, fairly, compassionately, justly, and more.

Thus, VE concerns itself with virtue as essential to achieving a good life. The virtues are character traits and practical intellect that are necessary for happiness. As Peter Geach famously pointed out, "Men need virtues as bees need stings."[29] The virtues give the right ends in the fulfillment of life and thus function as internal guides. For example, generosity makes us help others in need, and practical wisdom enables us to understand whether others are in real need of our help and how to go about helping them.[30]

Furthermore, VE takes a very distinctive approach to moral evaluation compared to deontology or utilitarianism. To use an illustration, in the Greek myth, Procrustes offered his bed to guests who wanted to spend the night. If the guests were too long, he would chop off their legs; if they were too short, he would stretch them to fit. The approaches of deontology and utilitarianism, in my view, are similar to what Procrustes used to do to his guests. VE, instead, understands morality by considering each situation, determining the appropriate moral approach, and thus which action should be carried out. Moreover, VE offers a practical way to live. It focuses on educating and developing into the kind of moral person who acquires the skill to make good moral deliberation. Becoming a just, moderate, compassionate person will enable one to do what is right, for the right reason, at the right time, in a given circumstance.

In Book II of the *Ethics*, Aristotle discusses the question of how one acquires the moral virtues, "the virtues . . . we acquire by having first put them into action."[31] For example, it is by repeatedly performing generous acts that one develops the virtue of generosity; it is by repeatedly refusing to indulge one's appetite that one develops the virtue of temperance. However, not every generous or temperate act is virtuous. If I spend my entire paycheck to buy a friend a car or if I refrain from eating altogether, or if I eat far too much, then I am not doing what is virtuous. Consider the virtue of courage. Being courageous is not lacking fear but acting in spite of fear. But if I express my courage by robbing a bank, I am not exercising my courage in a way that is virtuous. Why? Simply because robbing a bank is an action proceeding from a vice that goes against other virtues, such as justice. According to VE, the best way to promote social cooperation and harmony is for people to acquire a good, reliable character. Rules by themselves may give guidelines, but they cannot make people good. Consequences of our actions are important, but without good character we are not likely to produce greater total satisfaction that other theories try to achieve by detached theorizing.

Moral virtue involves intellectual excellence. VE argues that a virtuous individual has the ability to deliberate well and to see what is morally relevant in any particular situation. Another interesting criticism of VE is an argument proposed by Julia Driver. Driver proposes a consequentialist approach according to which virtue is a character trait conducive to good consequences. Her consequentialism is a version of objective consequentialism because it relies on actual consequences to determine the right course of action; it is also a type of evaluational externalism since factors external to an individual determine the moral goodness or badness of an act or an individual.

According to Driver, what VE refers to as the virtues are dispositions that promote social good, but they need not produce good consequences every time.[32] For Driver, an agent could be virtuous even without using the virtues or acknowledging them. Thus a virtue is a trait that "produces more good (in the actual world) than not systematically."[33] For example, a truly modest individual is one who (according to Driver) by definition underestimates his or her actual self-worth. Driver's aim is to challenge the classical conception of virtue, which requires that an agent have knowledge of relevant moral factors. She takes modesty in particular to be a "paradigm case of this type of virtue."[34] The modest person, according to Driver, cannot be modest and have accurate knowledge of his or her self-worth:

> What the analysis comes down to is this: for a person to be modest, she must be ignorant with regard to her self-worth. She must think herself less deserving, or less worthy, than she actually is. . . . Since modesty is generally considered to be a virtue, it would seem that this virtue rests upon an epistemic defect.[35]

Driver makes reference to the fact that a genuinely modest individual has a high regard of himself, but not as high as it in fact is. He underestimates his self-worth, but not to the point of self-deprecation. Driver writes, "The agent fails to fully recognize that, for example, he is the best pianist in the world when in fact he is."[36] Here she is in agreement with Bernard Williams that when a person acts virtuously, he or she does not do so because it is virtuous to act in such a way. And modesty fits this description because a modest person acts modestly without being aware that he or she is modest. Or, as Williams put it, "a modest person does not act under the title of modesty."[37] Similarly, a generous person acts generously, but not because he realizes that what he does is generous.[38] If that were the case, one would be falsely generous or falsely modest. Later, Driver also explains why we value modesty. We value modesty because a modest person "does not exhibit the vice of exaggeration." Thus, Driver considers modesty a virtue because the modest agent underestimates himself, and underestimation prevents being boastful or overranking "(e.g., an easing of tensions, lack of jealousies)."[39]

There are many problems with the account of modesty that Driver presents. Many commentators on modesty at this point have addressed these problems fairly thoroughly. Schueler offers an alternative account according to which a modest person has a lot to brag about, but he does not care whether others value these accomplishments highly.[40] By Schueler's account, modesty is compatible with having knowledge of one's abilities; one knows her abilities perfectly well, but is not interested in what others think about them. Some have pointed out that this account fails to recognize that the modest, after all, *would* care, at least in some respect, about the opinions of others. Allhoff, for example, argues that Schueler's account does not consider that "there are reasons other than being modest that might preclude someone from caring what others think about his accomplishments." In other words, it is possible that one "does not care" about what others think, but this nonchalant attitude might be due to being immodest.[41] Also, Bonmarito and Maes have noted that it seems incorrect to say that a modest person does not care about the opinions of others. Surely a great artist or athlete or benefactor who is modest may care about the praise and good reviews of others. There is nothing wrong with caring about the praise of others, I may add. Furthermore, not caring about the opinion of others would seem an example of immodesty.[42]

Furthermore, McMullin proposes instead that modesty involves an accurate assessment of one's worth combined with sensitivity to the feelings of others that prevents one from talking about it too much. She argues that previous accounts of modesty ignore (or mischaracterize) this other-regarding aspect of modesty:

> A fundamental characteristic of modesty, then, is the fact that it is not simply a *self*-regarding attitude, but is instead a profoundly *other*-regarding stance. Though it involves a heightened mode of self-awareness, it is a type of self-awareness which is accessible to me only through (a) recognition of how I am being experienced in the eyes of others, and (b) a desire to alleviate any suffering that this may cause.[43]

McMullin also argues that, paradoxically, in order to be modest, one must realize in what ways she surpasses others, so she can then act in such a way as to protect them from that knowledge:

> Modesty is not ignorance of the self or indifference to others but an orientation towards protecting another person from the hurtful lack or loss in feelings of self-worth that may arise from the experience of having a "lower rank." This orientation arises precisely in response to modest people's self-*knowledge* regarding where they stand in terms of social ranking. If one did not realize or care how one's accomplishments and successes might be painful to someone else, one would have no reason to seek to downplay them, but would, on the contrary, simply *enjoy* them.[44]

The foregoing are just a few of the most representative responses to Driver's original account of modesty as a virtue of ignorance. They are, I would like to add, adroit accounts of modesty. At any rate, I wonder whether they are accurate accounts of a character trait that we might consider a virtue.

According to Driver, modesty is an uninformed underestimation of one's moral worth; however, if an agent is really ignorant of her own moral worth, then there is no way of telling whether she is deprecating herself or being arrogant. But if at least some knowledge is required, since as Driver writes, a "modest person would still have to have a rather high opinion of herself, just not as high as she is entitled to have,"[45] why can't we just say that the agent has the correct opinion of herself? Her reply to this seems to be that such an account is contrary to our understanding of modesty because if one is modest, she cannot have a correct opinion of herself. But I think that the following is arguably a consistent account of modesty as a true virtue: Suppose Einstein is having a discussion with a group of people about mathematics. Arguably, if Einstein points out that his knowledge of mathematics is superior to the group's knowledge, one may say that Einstein is being immodest. According to Driver's account, Einstein, in this hypothetical scenario, would be modest if he did not admit to having a superior knowledge of math; but in such a case he would underestimate himself, and therefore he would be ignorant of his skills. But if modesty is a virtue, then it is correct to say that a modest individual is one who has the correct opinion of himself. In the Einstein example, the scientist knows perfectly well his great knowledge of mathematics, but, as a modest individual, he also understands that his being a mathematical genius does not give him license to be boastful. So it seems reasonable to say that the modest individual who has the correct opinion of himself but does not use it to elevate himself above others will avoid mentioning that he is in certain respects better or superior to others.

The reason any given trait is a virtue for Driver is that it "is conducive (more conducive than not) to the good. Modesty in particular is a virtue because the modest agent "underestimates himself, and this leads to some good that is valued by those he interacts with (e.g., an easing of tensions, lack of jealousies)."[46] The idea is that an individual who does not have a correct opinion and understanding of herself interacts with, for example, jealous people, so that her misunderstanding of her own character is supposed to ease tensions and cure one of jealousy. A genuine virtue eases tensions or avoids instances of jealousy, but most importantly educates the jealous to outgrow his jealousy and develop a noble character. In other words, Driver is right in saying that a modest person by being modest may give people fewer opportunities to be jealous. And she is right in saying that modesty is a trait that may produce more good than not. But she is wrong in saying that modesty is a virtue of ignorance because a modest individual is one who has a correct opinion of himself but is not boastful about it. Another interesting, though brief, example Driver gives of a "virtue of ignorance" is beauty. She says that "ignorance of one's own beauty is often said to enhance it."[47] But once again, it does not seem to me that ignorance of one's beauty is a virtue. In fact, a virtuous individual, I believe, would have knowledge of her beauty while at the same time she would know how unimportant being beautiful is. A great example that comes to mind is Socrates, who, arguably, knew that "no man is wiser than he," yet at the same time he understood that being wise or wiser or the wisest is not so important as to give one permission to be arrogant. So, modesty and beauty are useful utilitarian tools, but not virtues. My point here is that virtue does indeed require knowledge.

Driver also attacks Aristotelian virtue by arguing that virtue does not require good intentions or good motives. Her argument is a consideration of Huckleberry Finn saving his friend Jim from the slave hunters. She writes that Huck has "subjectively bad intentions and fails to know what the right thing to do is, yet his sympathetic heart warrants our commendation."[48] Huck's actions, however, are not—and cannot—be regarded as virtuous.

Huck does not think that slavery is an immoral institution that should be eliminated or anything along these lines. A virtuous person would. Strangely enough, Huck's best friend is a slave named Jim. When Jim runs away from his master, Huck does not turn him in. Now, what I find interesting is this. As Driver also notes, "Huckleberry also believes that this failure on his part [of not turning in Jim] is a moral failure—that he is, in effect, a party to the theft. He believes that what he is doing is dishonest and ungrateful."[49] But Huck's behavior is in no way virtuous. And I would even question whether his actions can be viewed as good or conducive to the good. In the first place, we have to wonder whether Huck saves Jim because he genuinely loves him or because he loves himself; that is, it might be argued that he saves Jim because he is interested in his relationship with Jim in a selfish sense—in the sense that he wants Jim as a friend and needs his company perhaps more than he is interested in what Jim wants.

What is clear to me is that there is something morally wrong with Huck. Namely, he does not condemn slavery, but he lets one slave run away. His actions stem from a possibly selfish desire to have his friend. In what sense are his actions promoting the good? Certainly it is not a bad thing to help a slave run away, though it is coincidental. But as to whether Huck's action can be considered virtuous or good in the sense of producing good for others, it is questionable. While Huck's action might help a particular slave—Jim—his attitude, especially his failure to connect the dots that Jim is no different from any other slave and thus slavery is immoral, is not necessarily conducive to the overall good. What if Huck had an argument with Jim (over who won a game, for instance)? Perhaps in that case he would resent Jim and feel less inclined to save him. And, arguably, Huck would not repeat the same gesture for any other slaves. So you can remove the requirement of knowledge and good intention from the concept of virtue, but only at the cost that you no longer deal with virtue, but rather with a form of utilitarianism.

As a result, the problem with Driver's consequentialist view is that it does not need to rely on the virtues at all. In fact, if knowledge and good motives are not required for an agent to be virtuous, then what we are talking about is simply utilitarianism, perhaps some elaborate form of act utilitarianism, because any action that happens to produce good consequences would be regarded as virtuous. The point of VE is that the agent acts out of a virtuous character and out of love for others. If I act solely to produce good consequences, I might be motivated only if I am in the pertinent psychological state; as in the case of Huck, I might want to act in a certain way not necessarily because I set out to produce good consequences, but only because I just happen to feel that way, perhaps for selfish reasons. And in fact Finn cannot be relied upon to save other slaves because he does not believe that slavery is immoral. When we apply Driver's account to the question of our obligations toward animals, we obtain unsatisfactory results. We go right back to the same problem—that we are supposed to become vegans because it produces good consequences. In the end, Driver's moral view turns out to be another example of a formula concerned about utility rather than relationships, care, and other factors that matter to us. As in the case of Huck, who does not understand why slavery is immoral, Driver's account of morality might suggest approaching the morality of our relationship with animals on the basis producing good consequences. As I have stressed this issue a number of times, consequentialism is not the correct way to approach the morality of our relationship with animals; the problem is that consequentialism, whether it is about preferences or rules, or whether it tries to accommodate the virtues, is still utilitarianism, and thus it simply is not reliable.

NOTES

1. I borrow this terminology from Anscombe to designate the moral theories derived from Kant, Bentham, Sidgwick, Moore, and other non-aretaic theories.
2. See Daniel C. Russell's "Virtue Ethics in Modern Moral Philosophy" and Dorothea Frede's "The Historic Decline of Virtue Ethics," in *The Cambridge Companion to Virtue Ethics* (Cambridge: Cambridge University Press, 2013).
3. Rosalind Hursthouse, *On Virtue Ethics* (Oxford: Oxford University Press, 1999), 47. See also a discussion by Liezl Van Zyl in "Virtue Ethics and Right Action," in *The Cambridge Companion to Virtue Ethics* (Cambridge: Cambridge University Press, 2013), 176–77.
4. Ibid., 28.
5. Aristotle, *Nichomachean Ethics* (Cambridge: Cambridge University Press, 2000). 1109a21f.
6. Ibid., III. 6–v.
7. Ibid., III. 10–12.
8. See Christine Swanton, "The Definition of Virtue Ethics," in *Cambridge Companion of Virtue Ethics* (Cambridge: Cambridge University Press, 2013), 315–338.
9. Hursthouse, *On Virtue Ethics*, 8.
10. Sinsheimer, "The Prospect of Designed Genetic Change," *Engineering and Science* 32, no. 7 (April 1969): 8–13.
11. Mary Midgley, "Biotechnology and Monstrosity: Why We Should Pay Attention to the 'Yuk Factor,'" *Hastings Center Report* 30, no. 5 (2000): 7–15.
12. John McDowell, "Two Sorts of Naturalism," in *Virtues and Reasons: Philippa Foot and Moral Theory: Essays in Honour of Philippa Foot*, ed. Rosalind Hursthouse, Gavin Lawrence, and Warren Quinn (Oxford: Oxford University Press, 1998), 153–155.
13. Immanuel Kant, *Critique of Pure Reason* (Cambridge: Cambridge University Press, 1998), A203/B248.
14. Midgley, "Biotechnology and Monstrosity," p. 8.
15. See John McDowell, "Two Sorts of Naturalism," 153–155.
16. Aristotle, *Nichomachean Ethics*, I. 2.
17. Ibid., I. 7.
18. Plato, *Euthyphro*, in *Five Dialogues: Euthyphro, Apology, Crito, Meno, Phaedo*, 2nd ed., ed. John M. Cooper and trans. G. M. A. Grube (Indianapolis: Hackett Publishing Company, 2002), 10a.
19. Hursthouse, *On Virtue Ethics*, 28.
20. Aristotle, *Nichomachean Ethics*, II. 6.
21. Ibid., III. 1.

22. For examples of agent-based theorists see Michael Slote, *Morals from Motives* (Oxford: Oxford University Press, 2001) and Linda Zagzebski, *Divine Motivation Theory* (New York: Cambridge University Press, 2004).

23. See Hursthouse, "Virtue Theory and Abortion," *Philosophy & Public Affairs* 20, no. 3 (1991): 223–246.

24. Plato, *Crito*, 48b.

25. J. L. Mackie, *Ethics: Inventing Right and Wrong* (New York: Penguin Books, 1977), 186.

26. Robert Louden, "Some Vices of Virtue Ethics," in *Ethical Theory Classic and Contemporary Readings*, (1st edition), ed. Louis Pojman (1989), 313–314.

27. See Hursthouse, "Virtue Theory and Abortion."

28. Aristotle, *Nichomachean Ethics*, I.7, I.13.

29. Peter Geach, *The Virtues: The Stanton Lectures 1973–74*, 1st edition (Cambridge: Cambridge University Press, 1977), 17.

30. Aristotle, *Nichomachean Ethics*, VI.I.2.

31. Ibid., II. 1103a30.

32. Julia Driver, *Uneasy Virtue* (Cambridge: Cambridge University Press, 2001), 74.

33. Ibid., 82.

34. Ibid., 16.

35. Ibid., 19.

36. Ibid., xvi.

37. Bernard Williams, *Ethics and the Limits of Philosophy* (Cambridge, MA: Harvard University Press, 1985), 10.

38. Driver, *Uneasy Virtue*, 10.

39. Ibid., 26.

40. G. F. Schueler, "Why Modesty Is a Virtue," *Ethics* 107, no. 3 (1997): 838.

41. Francis Allhoff, "What Is Modesty?" *International Journal of Applied Philosophy* 23, no. 2, (2010): 167.

42. Nicolas Bommarito, "Modesty as a Virtue of Attention," *Philosophical Review* 122, no. 1: 93–117, doi: 10.1215/00318108-1728723 (2013), 96.

43. Irene McMullin, "A Modest Proposal: Accounting for the Virtuousness of Modesty," *The Philosophical Quarterly* 60 (2010): 786.

44. McMullin, "A Modest Proposal," 787.

45. Driver, *Uneasy Virtue*, 19.

46. Ibid., 26.

47. Ibid., 28.

48. Ibid., 62.

49. Ibid., 52.

Chapter Five

What about Our Treatment of Animals?

As discussed, VE focuses on the development of the character of individuals and their flourishing. Some might wonder whether this means that human actions according to reason are necessary to achieve only human flourishing. In that case, VE has no resources to demonstrate that we have to be kind to animals. After all, Aristotle did not seem to have great things to say about animals. But this view does not seem to me to be correct. After all, humans are not the only things that can flourish.[1] Also, it is hard to imagine flourishing in an egotistic society. Furthermore, neglecting or not caring about others is precisely the opposite of how a virtuous person lives. Rebecca Walker, for example, argues that because others flourish like us, we have a reason to care about their flourishing as well. She points out that humans can extend this care to animals who, though not by definition virtuous or vicious, have needs and wants and characteristics that overlap with ours.[2] As discussed earlier, VE is a social practice. Unlike other theories, VE is primarily interested in the virtues and the way the virtues regulate emotion and human action in a way that is conducive to flourishing. Consequently, virtuous living harmonizes human existence with others and with nature. Whether things go well or badly for the virtuous individual depends on whether things go well or badly for everything that makes a good life possible, which includes other human beings but also animals and indeed the environment. It seems clear, then, that a direct concern for the good of animals can feature in VE. Therefore, I argue that a life lived well entails caring for non-human animals.

Chapter 5
THE SCOPE OF VIRTUE

VE addresses our treatment of animals in a very practical way. As Hursthouse argues, "Applying virtue ethics to moral issues should be straightforward. After all, it basically just amounts to thinking about what to do using the virtue and vice terms."[3] Precisely, if we are serious about morality, and our treatment of animals, we should want to treat them with respect as an expression of virtue. But apparently this position is not so straightforward. To mention one example, which I think exemplifies the general nature of this criticism, Tom Regan points out the danger of a theory whose principles are virtues. Although he is not exactly referring to virtue theory, it is worthwhile to consider what he has to say about an approach that he calls "the cruelty-kindness view."[4] This view says that we have to treat animals kindly and not be cruel to them. Regan argues, "Despite the familiar, reassuring ring of these ideas, I do not believe that this view offers an adequate theory."[5] Why does he find this view inadequate? When we consider kindness, he points out that a kind person acts out of compassion or concern or, as he says, out of virtue. But Regan laments that "there is no guarantee that a kind act is a right act."[6] In fact, he argues, one could be a kind racist, for example, who acts kindly toward members of his own race. Cruelty fares no better. Cruel people or their acts display either a lack of sympathy for or enjoyment in others' suffering. But while cruelty is bad, Regan writes, just as an agent's kindness does not guarantee that she does what is right, so the absence of cruelty does not guarantee that one will avoid performing a wrong act. Then Regan makes a statement that I find interesting. He says, "Many people who perform abortions, for example, are not cruel, sadistic people. But that fact alone does not settle the terribly difficult question of the morality of abortion."[7] If he says that people who perform abortions are not cruel and then that the question of the morality of abortion is not settled, then he begs the question. For he assumes that performing abortions is not a cruel act. He continues, "The case is no different when we examine the ethics of our treatment of animals. So, yes, let us be for kindness and against cruelty. But let us not suppose that being for the one and against the other answers questions about moral right and wrong."[8]

I disagree with Regan that being for kindness and against cruelty may not be enough as guidance to make us treat animals with respect. My response to this type of observation is that one must be kind in the full sense of it. If one is kind only to one's friends, then by definition he is not kind. By kindness I mean the quality of being friendly, considerate, and generous. One who is truly kind, therefore, would extend kindness indiscriminately. Also, according to VE, kindness intended as a virtue involves practical wisdom—that is, understanding of how to apply kindness. As Philippa Foot argues in *Natural Goodness*, "Goodness of choice or of will contains reason-recognition and following."[9] In fact, a virtuous agent recognizes reasons for action, ponders them, and responds appropriately to a given situation. The agent is motivated by, and acts in accordance with, one's virtuous character. The way we know what we should do depends on our nature such that right reasons derive from the facts about our human nature. Thus, facts and values are not separable.

In his review of Foot's *Natural Goodness*, Marc Murphy makes an interesting criticism. He discusses Foot's examples in which an anthropologist, Maklay, decides not to photograph a tribesman, despite having an opportunity to do so while the tribesman is asleep. In fact, Maklay promises not to take his photograph.[10] The point here is that the tribesman does not want to be photographed for superstitious reasons, and Maklay is aware of that. So, considering that such photographs might bring knowledge to society about the life of certain tribes, and considering that the tribesman is sleeping, why not take the photograph after all? Murphy writes,

> Given that the disposition to trustworthiness is good for human beings, so that a person without that disposition is defective in some way, how can we show that the act of photographing the tribesman was itself defective, a bad act? Foot's argument moves in a large, lazy circle here.[11]

I am not sure why Murphy sees a "lazy circle" here. I'm surprised that he cannot see why photographing the tribesman is wrong. Perhaps Murphy, like many other critics who advance similar points, has been disciplined by utilitarian ideas and thinks that taking the photograph would not, after all, do any wrong to the tribesman; it wouldn't hurt him physically or spiritually, and because he was sleeping, he wouldn't feel disrespected. But the very point of VE is that Maklay would do what is right because it conforms to the character of a virtuous person—that is, a person who has the virtue of trustworthiness.

In other words, what a virtuous ethicist sees that Murphy misses is that Maklay promised the tribesman not to take any photographs of him. In promising this, Maklay is in a very important sense also making a personal commitment, a promise to himself. He is committing to keeping a promise. He is saying to himself, "I recognize and accept that to take such a photograph would be wrong because it betrays the tribesman," so by taking the photo he would wrong the tribesman—but most importantly, he would betray himself by resorting to lying or not keeping his promise. So if he took the opportunity to take the photo while the tribesman slept, Maklay would disrespect himself by behaving irrationally, first by making a promise to himself and the tribesman and then by breaking it.

Simply put, a virtuous agent is kind and against cruelty and his or her actions are actions of love. By this definition, considering that animals are killed to satisfy the taste for meat, a virtuous individual's nature is contrary to treating animals as property and regarding them as food. It is clear that one cannot be a kind individual and at the same time feed on the flesh of a dead animal. The example of the supposedly kind racist is a distortion of VE or of virtues. Just as one does not possess the virtue of courage for having the guts to rob a bank, so a racist does not perform a kind, virtuous act for being kind to a member of the same race while unkind to members of another race. Similarly, as Augustine said, if I love others, by definition I care about their well-being. And to say, for example, that love does not guarantee that I do what is right because, for example, one may love to murder, is a distortion of the meaning of love:

> What does love look like? It has the hands to help others. It has the feet to hasten to the poor and needy. It has eyes to see misery and want. It has the ears to hear the sighs and sorrows of men. That is what love looks like.[12]

When we pause to reflect on the pain people inflict upon animals, it is hard to see how utilitarians and deontologists (or rights theorists) actually propose that we should respect animals on the basis of rights, duty, or maximum utility. That's not why we should respect animals. VE proposes that we understand the importance of all life. As Gordon Preece writes, "Though beech trees feel no pain, they may be morally significant; because of what they are created to be, they shouldn't be chopped down indiscriminately."[13] The approach I argue for here is that a viable animal ethics should embrace the intrinsic value of all life, whether human, animal, or biosphere. Deontological and utilitarian theories cannot capture the importance of our moral experience. These theories force us to understand our relationship with animals in terms of duty, right, or utility. But the value of creatures cannot be put into those terms.

It is a fact, however, that those theories have shaped our understanding of the human/animal relationship. Those approaches seem to create moral inconsistencies. A salient illustration of this is a YouTube video showing a man in a supermarket pretending to be a butcher who promotes a certain brand of sausages.[14] He cooks the sausages and gives samples to shoppers, many of whom compliment him for the great taste and freshness of his product. When some of them decide to buy the sausages, the "butcher" pulls a piglet out of a box and drops it into what seems to be meat grinder—that is the secret behind the freshness of his sausages. At this point the reaction of practically all shoppers is the same—they're shocked by the cruel death that the "butcher" is about to inflict on that poor piglet. They are appalled by his indifference and protest that the piglet be left alone and allowed to live. What is curious about this social experiment is that at this point most of the customers are still chewing on their sausage! This reminds me of a passage in Mary Midgley's article, "Biotechnology and Monstrosity" where Midgley says: "It is especially unfortunate that people often now have the impression that while feeling is against them, reason quite simply favors the new developments."[15] Here Midgley discusses the emotional reaction of people to biotechnology. Her point is that these sorts of reactions are typically discounted as merely emotional, but in fact they constitute an important component of morality. Granted, emotions are not infallible; but it is a mistake to forthright dismiss them as "just emotions." These emotions often are pre-rational, but not irrational, reasons. I think the YouTube video I am referring to should give us pause. Such reactions evince what I think is a natural, compassionate response to a callous and unjust act. Unfortunately, our natural feeling of compassion is taken over by other factors. This is something that Timothy Pachirat describes at length in *Every Twelve Seconds*. In chapter 1, he discusses the idea that I am trying to convey by saying that "contemporary, industrialized slaughter . . . distance and concealment operate as mechanism of power in modern society."[16] In other words, while we recognize the intrinsic value and beauty of animals, we are taught not to rely on this feeling, but rather on the practicality of meat production and consumption. I don't find it surprising that this moral blindness is due to an ethical view that seldom gives any thought to what the practice of eating animals says about our moral character.

ANIMAL ETHICS NEEDS VIRTUE

For these reasons and more, a number of contemporary philosophers have suggested that an animal ethics should be framed in terms of virtuous character and acquiring the virtues, instead of trying to understand duty or utility or rights.[17] My suggestion is that the correct conception of morality is a virtue-oriented approach, and such an approach can make sense and show the correct attitude toward animals. Consequently, VE can show what is virtuous about ethical veganism. Shafer-Landau, for example, points out that the arguments about vegetarianism or veganism based on deontic or utilitarian defenses at best favor the abolition of factory farming, but still "this leaves us short of a moral obligation to remain or become vegetarians."[18] After all, the so-called Singer-Regan argument typically focuses on the immorality of factory farming. Singer himself is not a vegan, though Regan was. What factory farming does to animals is immoral, and that's agreed upon by most sensible people. But what about animals outside farms? Shafer-Landau suggests that perhaps we should abandon deontic and utilitarian concepts and instead focus on certain traits of character showing that the practices of using animals for food are typically callous. I say "typically" referring to what McPherson calls modest ethical veganism, "the view that it is typically morally wrong to use or eat products made from or by" animals such as cows, pigs, chickens, or fish, or products such as dairy and eggs.[19] Modest ethical veganism does not deem immoral any and all circumstances in which animals or animal by-products are used. Rather, it maintains that it is immoral to use animals when equal or superior plant-based alternatives are readily available, which is the case for most affluent societies. However, I am not suggesting that eating animals is a neutral act. To be clear, I think that eating an animal, her eggs, using her skin or pelt, or any other form of exploitation is wrong. By wrong I mean that all forms of animal exploitation are wrong because they are contrary to virtue (as I shall illustrate later).

Rosalind Hursthouse is a proponent of a virtuous approach to the ethical treatment of non-human animals. She argues that starting with the question of moral status, whether animals and humans are equal in some moral respect, or whether animals have rights, is not the correct starting point. Rather, we should begin by morally questioning the attitudes that underlie the use of animals. When we do so, we often find that we act viciously. Thus, if one is committed to living a virtuous life, he or she will change his or her attitude toward the use of animals.[20] Cheryl Abbate also entertains the idea that virtue ethics, rather than utilitarianism or duty or rights view, is the appropriate framework for developing a defense of ethical veganism. Her claim is that on the one hand, utilitarianism is overly permissive because it permits the harming of animals for trivial reasons, so long as aggregate utility is maximized. On the other hand, deontological theory is too restrictive, since the prohibition on harming nonhuman animals would make moral agents incapable of responding to moral tragedies that, at times, may require that some animals be harmed in order to prevent more harm.[21] Furthermore, Brian Luke argues that the most influential arguments in favor of veganism or vegetarianism (especially those proposed by Regan and Singer) rely on conceptions of rights and preference that are flawed. Both Regan and Singer, though they propose different ethical accounts, share the idea that there is no morally relevant difference between animals and humans that could justify animal exploitation. So, Regan argues that because animals are "subjects-of-a-life" like humans, in the sense that they feel and have desires and a variety of experiences just like us, and because they can be harmed just like humans, they also have a value that should be respected. The difficulty with these types of arguments is that the symmetry they propose between human and non-human animals is questionable. In fact, it may be argued that it is an example of anthropomorphism to say that our experiences are similar to those of certain animals in a way that is relevant to morality. As mentioned earlier, Peter Singer clearly defends the notion that it is not inherently immoral to kill an animal because animals do not have an understanding of continuous self. Many others hold a similar position. Michael Tooley, for example, argues that it is not immoral to kill most animals because they are not cognitively sophisticated enough to have a concept of continued existence. So, depriving them of their future is not wrong as it is to deprive a human being who is aware of and cares about his continued existence.[22] Furthermore, as Carl Cohen argues, not all suffering is equal, and human suffering, and human pleasure, are much more important than animal suffering (or pleasure).[23] The problem with assuming such a symmetry is that since the cognitive capacities of animals are not sophisticated enough, and their suffering, it is suggested, is not as important as human suffering, it is not wrong, for example, to kill them in ways that cause minimal suffering.[24]

Thus, VE has a great deal to say about animal ethics. And I think it has a lot to say about ethical veganism. I find it surprising that not enough virtue ethicists are clearly interested in ethical veganism. VE is the view that humanity has a final goal—happiness—and to fulfill this goal it is necessary to develop a sound, moral character, a character guided by the virtues. Another way to put it is that a human being without virtue is defective. A good human being is sensitive to the suffering of others, against injustice, and temperate regarding food. Consequently, it is difficult to see how one could defend a virtue-based viewpoint in line with any form of animal exploitation. What is interesting to note is that, in fact, no virtuous ethicist, as far as I know, has ever proposed that eating meat is consistent with being virtuous. Nevertheless, I don't doubt that some may think it would be possible. In considering this, it is important to note at least two points: animals are not food. This is obviously a point of contention. Since animals have been eaten for millennia, some may ask, "Why are they not food?" I want to propose that animals are not food for the same reason that humans are not food. Aristotle said that the function of human beings is rational activity. Human good, therefore, is rational activity performed well, which means in accordance with virtue. This is the so-called Function Argument, which has been widely criticized. I find most criticisms to be wrongheaded because they try to read too much into the term "function." In a very practical way (which is what I think Aristotle wanted to achieve by proposing this notion) "function" does not mean purpose in the sense that humans were designed, as it were, for a function just like knives and computers. Rather, a way of understanding "function" is simply "how a thing does what it does." As Korsgaard notes,

> So when Aristotle says that the function of a human being is the activity of the rational part of the soul, he does not mean simply that reasoning is the purpose of a human being. Nor does he mean merely that it is a characteristic activity of human beings, if we understand that to mean only that it is an activity which, as it happens, picks out the species uniquely. He means rather that rational activity is how we human beings do what we do, and in particular, how we lead our specific form of life.[25]

And thus what is characteristic about human beings is that they do things by making rational choices. This is, in my view, an observation that could easily be made by some aliens visiting our planet. In inspecting a mango and a human being, I find it hard to believe that any creature endowed with reason could possibly believe that the function of both objects is to be food. An intelligent alien would arguably realize that humans make rational choices that are conducive to some sort of life-fulfillment activity. They would realize that humans have projects, make children, that they learn a variety of concepts, that they are social individuals, and so on. But what they would not see is that humans are food. My point is, then, that the same rationale applies to animals. Animals are not food in this sense in that they exist for their own benefit. The second point is a simple one that will no doubt raise lots of questions. At any rate, in the same sense that I use the word "function" to describe human beings (not in the sense that humans were designed, perhaps by God, to have a specific function), I want to suggest that there are biological facts indicating that human food is fruit and vegetables—not meat or animal products. It is often said that human beings are omnivores. But it seems to me that an omnivore is a creature that could thrive either on an exclusively meat-based diet or an exclusively plant-based diet. However, while human beings can thrive on an exclusive plant-based diet, they cannot survive on an exclusive meat-based diet. One of the reasons is that humans cannot synthesize vitamin C, among others micronutrients.[26] Carnivores, on the other hand, can. Scurvy occurs in humans as a result of not getting enough vitamin C; but no carnivorous animals ever got scurvy, because their bodies synthesize the vitamin. Also, human beings can synthesize taurine, a sulfur-containing amino acid important in the metabolism of fats, while carnivores cannot. This is not surprising considering that carnivores are not "designed" by nature to eat fruits and vegetables, but rather meat. Conversely, humans synthesize taurine but must consume vegetables and fruit to acquire vitamin C.[27] I would like to note that my argument here is not that humans are obligated to eat plants and fruit because plants and fruit constitute natural human food. Rather, my point is that because humans have a natural food, consuming that food is conducive to flourishing.

Furthermore, our relationship with animals is a relationship of power. Humans have domesticated many animals and benefited from them, while animals are harmed. But to be indifferent to the facts just mentioned and to the harm that animals suffer when killed for food, whether by ourselves or by others, can hardly be considered an attitude that qualifies an individual as virtuous. As I have pointed out, to be virtuous means to fulfill our potential to flourish. But this is not possible to achieve, as it were, in a vacuum. Success in fulfilling this end is also predicated upon our relationship with others, and consequently by letting others fulfill their ends as well. Since sentient beings are harmed when they cannot satisfy their own best interests, the virtue ethics approach implies respecting the interests of others. Moreover, because insensitivity is not considered virtuous, but compassion and care are, it follows that a virtuous person would not only refrain from harming animals, but also do good and try to help them whenever possible.

NOTES

1. Julia Annas made the same point. See *The Morality of Happiness* (Oxford: Oxford University Press, 1993), especially pp. 127–128, 223, 322–325.
2. Rebecca Walker, "The Good Life for Non-Human Animals: What Virtue Requires of Humans," in *Working Virtue*, ed. Rebecca L. Walker and Philip J. Ivanhoe (Oxford: Oxford University Press, 2007), 173–90.
3. Hursthouse, "Applying Virtue Ethics on the Treatment of the Other Animals," 136.
4. Tom Regan, "The Case for Animal Rights," in Peter Singer (ed.), *In Defense of Animals* (1985), 13–26.
5. Ibid., 16.
6. Ibid., 16.
7. Ibid., 16.
8. Ibid., 16.
9. Philippa Foot, *Natural Goodness* (Oxford: Clarendon Press, 2001), 13.
10. Ibid., 47.
11. Marc Murphy, "Book Review," *Ethics* 113, no. 2 (January 2003): 411.
12. St. Augustine, *Confessions*, as quoted in *Quote, Unquote*, ed. Lloyd Cory (Victor Books, 1977), 197.
13. Preece, "The Unthinkable & Unbelievable Singer," 44.
14. There are several similar videos on YouTube. This particular one is "Brazilian Pig Eating Prank," https://www.youtube.com/watch?v=oL-UAMzFqEM, published on June 26, 2014, by VeganRevolution.
15. Midgley, "Biotechnology and Monstrosity," 8.
16. Timothy Pachirat, *Every Twelve Seconds: Industrialized Slaughter and the Politics of Sight* (New Haven, CT: Yale University Press, 2013).
17. Utilitarians and deontologists have been the dominant forces in the recent literature on ethical issues regarding animals. The literature is vast, but the most influential are the works of Peter Singer and Tom Regan: Tom Regan, *The Case for Animal Rights*, rev. ed. (Berkeley: University of California Press, 2004); Peter Singer, *Animal Liberation: A New Ethics for Our Treatment of Animals* (New York: Avon Books, 1975); Peter Singer, *Practical Ethics*, 2nd ed. (Cambridge: Cambridge University Press, 1993); and Peter Singer, "Utilitarianism and Vegetarianism," *Philosophy and Public Affairs* 9, no. 4 (1980): 305–324.
18. Shafer-Landau, "Vegetarianism, Causation and Ethical Theory," *Public Affairs Quarterly* 8, no. 1 (January 1994).
19. Tristram McPherson, "Why I Am a Vegan (and You Should Be One Too)," in *Philosophy Comes to Dinner* (Abingdon, UK: Routledge, 2015), 73–91.
20. See Hursthouse, *On Virtue Ethics* (Oxford: Oxford University Press, 1999); R. Hursthouse, "Applying Virtue Ethics to Our Treatment of Other Animals," in *The Practice of Virtue: Classic and Contemporary Readings in Virtue Ethics*, ed. J. Welchman (Indianapolis: Hackett Publishing, 2006); R. Hursthouse, "Virtue Ethics and the Treatment of Animals," in *The Oxford Handbook of Animal Ethics*, ed. T. Beauchamp and R. Frey (Oxford: Oxford University Press, 2011).
21. Cheryl Abbate, "Virtues and Animals: A Minimally Decent Ethic for Practical Living in a Non-Ideal World," *Journal of Agricultural and Environmental Ethics* 27, no. 6 (2014): 909–929.
22. Michael Tooley, "Abortion and Infanticide," *Philosophy and Public Affairs* 2, no. 1 (1972): 37–65.
23. Carl Cohen, "The Case for the Use of Animals in Biomedical Research," *The New England Journal of Medicine* 315 (1986): 865–869.

24. Brian Luke, "Justice, Caring and Animal Liberation," in *The Feminist Care Tradition in Animal Ethics: A Reader* (New York: Columbia University Press, 2007), 124–148.

25. Korsgaard, "Fellow Creatures," 141.

26. G. Drouin, J. R. Godin, and B. Pagé, "The Genetics of Vitamin C Loss in Vertebrates," doi:10.2174/138920211796429736.

27. W. C. Roberts, "Twenty Questions on Atherosclerosis," *Proceedings* (Baylor University Medical Center) 13, no. 2 (2000): 139–143.

Chapter Six

Veganism as a Virtue

EMBRACING VIRTUE

Having considered some of the most telling shortcomings of the ethics of duty and the ethics of consequences, it is no surprise that in recent years, moral philosophy has seen a revival of virtue ethics.[1] It is natural that many moral philosophers felt the need to return to a theory of morality that is in tune with human nature. Consequentialism and deontology, as we have seen, can be described with one word: detached. Consequently, moral thinkers recently rediscovered VE due to its emphasis on "moral education, moral wisdom and discernment, friendship and family relationships, a deep concern of happiness, the role of emotions in our moral life, and the question of what sort of person I should be, and how we should live."[2] Incidentally (or perhaps not), some moral philosophers have expressed interest in ethical veganism. The point that I have been trying to allude to all along here is that moral thinking will benefit greatly from virtue ethics. When we think in terms of virtue, we make sense of many aspects of morality that are concealed or untouched questions of duty. For example, this is very clear from my earlier discussion on Kant's indirect duty toward animals. Kant sought to determine our duty toward animals by leaving out many important aspects of the same question—namely, relationship, feeling, and human and animal nature. As I pointed out, Kant's strategy does not work. Surely Kant demonstrates what reason instructs us to do. Kant showed that acting rightly is equivalent to acting rationally. But his tunnel vision makes it impossible to see that disrespecting an animal is intrinsically callous.

Virtue ethics is constantly under attack for many reasons: How exactly are virtues measures, reliable, applied, etc.? These, and many others, are theoretical issues that need to be worked out by normative ethicists and need not be a worry in the present discussion. What is important is to see what kind of suggestions a virtue ethics is capable of giving. And I think that a virtuous approach to morality, specifically regarding animal ethics, can be used in support of ethical veganism. One wonders why virtue ethicists seldom have contemplated this prospect. Ethical veganism, essentially, is the ideal of categorically abolishing animal exploitation. This ideal amounts to saying that using animals or insects as a source of food, clothing, scientific research, and more is immoral. This position is sometimes referred to as absolute veganism. Over the years of thinking and arguing for this position, many have pointed out to me that it is difficult, if not impossible, to justify such a totalizing claim in the face of, for example, those who live in parts of the world where scarcity of plant food or other unfavorable factors leave them with no other choice but to use animals to survive. Furthermore, avoiding products obtained from animals or that have been experimented on animals is nearly impossible since almost everything has been, including soya beans and even water. These objections are legitimate. However, it seems to me that they are mistaken for the following reason. Consider the now favorite example of moral philosophers: slavery. Surely it is an immoral institution, regardless of economic or other concerns. Similarly, if exploiting animals is an immoral practice, as I argue, the fact that the use of animals is so prominent does not mean that it is essential and unreplaceable. Granted, almost everything involves animal testing, even water. But it doesn't follow that it is right to do so. It does not follow, thus, that absolute veganism is an untenable position.

Consequently, a less radical view of veganism is proposed, though in my view it is not radical enough. For example, People for the Ethical Treatment of Animals (PETA) states, "We would not oppose eating eggs from chickens treated as companions if the birds receive excellent care and are not purchased from hatcheries."[3] This strikes me as a very peculiar form of veganism. Many vegans (including myself) would not eat eggs—even from chickens treated as companions. This is why I suggest looking at the issue from the point of view of virtue. A virtuous person, in my view, does not eat animals or animal parts at all. Having the virtue of temperance, for example, one eats what is conducive to health and what is necessary. Because eggs are not essential in a healthful diet, the virtuous person avoids eggs. Most importantly, eggs are the unfertilized reproductive cycles of chickens; they are not food. A virtuous person, it seems to me, is not one who seeks to eat animals or their secretions. Animals can in many cases be friends. Thus, it seems difficult to see how a virtuous person could eat the eggs or meat of a friend.

Ethical veganism often seems to be framed in terms derived from theories that I reject, theories that avail themselves of concepts of duty or utility. For example, as defined by the Vegan Society, veganism is best understood as "a philosophy and way of living which seeks to exclude—as far as is possible and practicable—all forms of exploitation of, and cruelty to, animals for food, clothing or any other purpose; and by extension, promotes the development and use of animal-free alternatives for the benefit of humans, animals and the environment."[4] But what is the ethical basis for excluding all forms of animal exploitation? Some define veganism as "the practice of minimizing harm to all animals, which requires abstention from animal products, such as meat, fish, dairy, eggs, honey, gelatin, lanolin, wool, fur, silk, suede and leather."[5] While it is reasonable to say that we can only hope to minimize harm inflicted on animals, we should not become ethical vegans only because it may minimize harm. I also worry that "requiring abstention" from animal products may be the wrong moral attitude. Abstention sounds like a diet. Diets are seldom successful because they ask one to abstain from what always turns out to be one's favorite food. I find this to be the wrong attitude. These approaches to ethical veganism are vaguely based on flawed utilitarian or deontic concepts suggesting that, as a rule, we abstain from using animals or, as a utilitarian principle, we do what minimizes undesirable consequences.

I am not arguing that minimizing suffering is not important; it obviously is, and so is avoiding animal products. Part of the solution, I argue, is to consider the individual moral character, which is what VE is all about, after all. Far from playing down the importance of reducing suffering, I am suggesting that perhaps it is time to worry about our moral character. "What kind of person should I be?" and "How should I live my life?" are questions that should feature in an animal ethics. My argument is based on virtue. I argue that a more conducive defense of ethical veganism is to consider ethical veganism an expression of virtuous character. While I agree with utilitarians that sentience is an important moral factor, I argue that in order to make sense of our relationship with animals we must first understand what it is to be a good individual. I believe that conducting a virtuous life leads to practicing veganism, not as an abstention or an attempt to maximize utility, but rather as an expression of good moral character, of what Aristotle calls "greatness of soul."[6]

SOME TENETS OF VIRTUE ETHICS

Considering that deontic and utilitarian arguments defending the moral obligation to become vegetarians or vegans are flawed, I shall discuss how virtue ethics can offer a more helpful approach. As many virtue ethicists point out, VE concerns itself with moral education and moral feelings, and thus maintains that our moral experience and our relationships with others are too complex, too nuanced, and too textured to be captured and understood by a set of principles or rational calculation. As illustrated earlier in the actual case of Singer's mother,[7] when we theorize, we detach ourselves from our moral experience and our moral feelings, overlooking the importance of our relationship with others and the importance of "sympathy, empathy, and compassion as relevant ethical and epistemological sources for human treatment of nonhuman animals."[8]

FOUR IMPORTANT VIRTUES: TEMPERANCE, COMPASSION, FAIRNESS, AND GREATNESS OF THE SOUL

In order to see in what sense ethical veganism may be an expression of virtue, it is helpful to consider some important aspects of the virtues of temperance, compassion, fairness, and also of what Aristotle calls greatness of the soul. These traits of character are epistemologically important to our understanding of our relationship with animals. They bring into light certain aspects of nature that other moral approaches discount. Virtues in my view make their possessor a good human being. As I suggested, all living things have a certain function or nature, and they can flourish. Our nature as human beings is to use reason. It is in our nature to act rationally, by virtue of which we make moral decisions. Acting virtuously thus means acting in accordance with reason, which is essential to achieve happiness. This means that the virtues directly benefit their possessor. And since human nature is social, acting virtuously is exercised in opposition to self-interest. Consequently, concern about all forms of life is essential to flourishing. And it is not just that the virtues enable us to achieve happiness; rather, a virtuous life is itself the good life because the exercise of our rational capacities and virtue is its own reward.

As an illustration, consider the unfortunate life events of Bernard L. Madoff and Steven Goff, two very different individuals. Madoff is an American former stockbroker, responsible for the largest Ponzi scheme in world history and the largest financial fraud in U.S. history. It is estimated that he defrauded investors out of approximately $65 billion. After his multibillion-dollar Ponzi scheme was uncovered, both he and his wife tried to commit suicide, as his wife declared to the press, "I don't know whose idea it was, but we decided to kill ourselves because it was so horrendous what was happening."[9] In the end, Madoff and his wife did not have the courage to do it, but their son, Mark Madoff, apparently out of shame for his father's actions, took his life by hanging himself with a dog leash.[10] Steven Goff, unlike Madoff, is a regular man, a former mechanic from Ventnor, New Jersey. In 2013, he confessed to murdering a fifteen-year-old, Frederick Hart, in May 1990. Goff told the victim's family, "I wanted to give you your justice. You deserve to see me suffer."[11] I think Madoff and Goff can serve as a perfect illustration of how a vicious life is itself devastating. Their predicaments remind us of the discussion in book IV of Plato's *Republic* about whether it is worth being just regardless of one's type of life. According to Socrates, individual injustice stems from the dis-order of the three parts of the soul. That is, the human soul according to Socrates is composed of three parts, which he labels the appetitive, the spirited, and the rational. A just individual is one whose rational part rules over the spirited and the appetitive; that is, each part performs its proper function according to nature and thus it is in the nature of reason to rule an individual's soul. Conversely, an unjust individual is one whose parts of the soul are not ordered according to nature. Any combination where reason is subordinate produces an unjust individual. Thus, for Socrates it is always worth being a just person despite appearance, because justice is, as it were, the health of one's soul. Glaucon acknowledges that

> even if one has every kind of food and drink, lots of money, and every sort of power to rule, life is thought not to be lived if the nature of the body is ruined. So if someone can do whatever he wishes, except what will free him from vice and injustice and make him have justice and virtue, how can it be worth living if the nature by which we live is ruined and in turmoil.[12]

While I am not necessarily endorsing Plato's tripartite theory of soul, Socrates' insight is very telling. It is not possible for an individual to live well when his or her life is ruined by vice, and the cases of Goff and Madoff, I believe, are an illustration of this. A life of virtue is ultimately desirable for its own sake and for the consequences. Madoff and Goff arguably could have continued living their lives and might never have been found out. Goff is not a multi-billionaire; Madoff was. But money or reputation or anything else would not have given these individuals happiness. My point then is that the virtues are necessary for a happy life, and vice always leads to a disgraceful life, though in various forms and degrees.

Aristotle defines each moral virtue in terms of action and emotion. Courage is defined in terms of our response to the fear we experience when we face a dangerous situation. Temperance is defined in terms of our response to desires for different pleasures. Why are moral virtues important? They are important so that we can know ourselves. The sort of self-knowledge that is acquired through the virtues is emotional self-awareness. Certainly it is difficult to acquire because it requires a life of practice and moral growth of each individual. VE suggests that the individual alone, through practical reasoning and virtuous action, must come to know himself or herself and the deeper subtleties of his or her emotional responses to circumstances.

The virtues should be considered in relation to what is known as the doctrine of the mean. In Book II of the *Ethics*, Aristotle discusses the notion of virtues as means between two extremes, one of excess one of defect. There he writes to consider that the excellence of a thing is that which makes it function properly. The excellence of an eye, for example, makes the eye good and enables it to function well as an eye. Likewise, the excellence of human beings is a disposition that makes humans good and enables them to perform their function well.[13] This function of human beings is "a way of living . . . consisting in the exercise of the psyche's capacities in accordance with reason, or at any rate not in opposition to reason." A good individual "exercises these capacities and performs these activities well." Thus, the best life for a human being involves "the active exercise of his psyche's capacities in accordance with excellence."[14] And in Book II, chapter 6, Aristotle defines excellence as "a settled disposition determining choice, involving the observance of the mean relative to us, this being determined by reason, as the practically wise person would determine it."[15] The notion of the mean for Aristotle is very simple. Health, for example, is destroyed by excess and deficiency. Too much food, or unhealthful food, or too much exercise or too little food are bad for health. The same principle holds in ethical matters. That is, excellence of character is destroyed by excess and deficiency.[16] Bodily health is a matter of observing a mean between extremes of excess and deficiency. Aristotle noted that excellence of character is concerned with emotions and acts, which can be excessive or deficient or moderate. For example, one can be scared or brave, feel desire or anger or pity, and experience pleasure and pain, either more or less than is right. However, having these feelings in moderation is a mark of excellence. Precisely, one should have such feelings at the right time, on the right occasion, toward the right people, for the right purpose, and in the right amount. Thus excellence is a mean state in the sense that it aims at the mean.

What happens when one's feelings are not moderate? Consider temperance. Temperance lies in a mean between the extremes of excessive and deficient enjoyment of sensual pleasures. For instance, one who enjoys too much food or enjoys food that is not necessary for good health but tastes or smells good (to that individual) is not temperate. The other extreme would be deficiency of such pleasures. For example, one who starves himself to the point of becoming ill is not a temperate individual. I have to note that the mean for Aristotle is "not of the thing itself but relative to us."[17] But "relative" here is not meant in the sense that two virtuous individuals would act in two completely different ways. Here Aristotle talks about how the amount of food for different individuals may vary, and consequently the amount of food required by an athlete would not be the same as that required by a sedentary person. Thus, not being moderate, not hitting the mean, leads to defect.

Aristotle discusses temperance and intemperance in Book III of the *Ethics* in terms of bodily pleasure and pain. The intemperate person, Aristotle argues, enjoys "the smells of perfumes and cooked dishes."[18] He describes intemperance as indulging in pleasures that are "slavish or brutish."[19] Temperance regulates our responses to appetite, which are very basic animal impulses.

With regard to eating, Aristotle noted that too much or too little will ruin one's health. He argued that "to eat whatever is at hand"[20] is a sign of intemperance. As stated earlier, temperance is not only about eating the right amount of food but also eating what is proper—that is, not whatever is available. A temperate individual, according to this characterization, eats food that is conducive to health, and in moderation, "as long as they are not incompatible with health or vigor, contrary with what is noble, or beyond his means."[21] Here Aristotle gives important insight. Being temperate means eating what is healthful, what is noble, and what is within one's means. The temperate individual thus is not attracted to any kind of food just because it smells or tastes good. Rather, he or she will eat in moderation, not to satisfy one's fancy, but to be nourished; thus food is what is healthful. Furthermore, what is noble seems to be related to what is within one's means. I take it to mean that food should not be an object of worship, so to speak. One should approach food in a modest manner. Food should not be extravagant and expensive, for example; rather, it should be simple, tasty, and nutritious. Also, the noble approach to food is to consume food that does not require harm to others and the environment, among other things.

From this consideration of what it is to be temperate, as it applies to healthful eating, I believe that considering animals as food evinces lack of temperance. In fact, by showing that eating animal products is unhealthful, it seems consistent to say that consuming animal products is immoral as it is an expression of the vice of intemperance. This consideration differs from the typical defenses of ethical veganism, as noted earlier, because it focuses on the individual rather than on the animals. That is to say, eating animals is disgraceful or wrong because it is an expression of excess. Again, I am not arguing that only character is important and animals themselves are not important. Animals are indeed important individuals, as I shall discuss later, and thus should be taken into consideration. When the idea of ethical veganism is considered by many, the typical wrong objection is that eating animals is after all a requirement. But this is demonstrably false. What is important here is to consider that it is not only possible to thrive on a vegan diet, a diet completely devoid of animal products, but also recommended. For many years now, health sciences have consistently shown that consuming animal products can be dangerous for one's health.[22] Scientific research is overwhelmingly positive that eating meat and dairy products can cause heart disease, diabetes, obesity, atherosclerosis formation, cancer, and other health issues; on the other hand, a plant-based diet may lower, and in many cases even reverse, those conditions.[23]

I always return to Midgley's point that certain acts are "themselves expression of disrespect . . . and naturally call for more of the same."[24] Here she points out that there is a connection between a bad act and its consequences. One cannot expect to act any kind of way without certain consequences. I find that eating animals is a mark of a defect of character, the consequences of which should be expected. Namely, it is not an accident that lack of temperance leads to eating animals and in turn leads to health problems. As a way of connecting temperance and veganism, I want to consider a few examples.

Cancer. In 2015, twenty-two scientists from the World Health Organization's International Agency for Research on Cancer evaluated over eight hundred medical studies and concluded that consumption of processed meat is "carcinogenic to humans," and that consumption of red meat is "probably carcinogenic to humans." Their conclusions were based on overwhelming evidence for positive associations between meat and colorectal cancer, as well as positive associations between processed meat consumption and stomach cancer, and between red meat consumption and pancreatic and prostate cancer. Furthermore, it is not just processed meats that can cause such health risks. The study also shows consumption of all kinds of animals, including "white meat," beef, pork, etc. can cause cancer.[25] According to Cancer Council of New South Wales, "There is now a clear body of evidence that bowel cancer is more common among those who eat the most red and processed meat." Also note that "meat may affect cancer risk because of chemicals formed during digestion that have been found to damage the cells that line the bowel."[26] As Casey Dunlop of Cancer Research UK notes, "a link between certain types of meat and some forms of cancer—notably bowel cancer—isn't 'new' news—the evidence has been building for decades, and is supported by a lot of careful research." And to quote Dr. Neal Bernard, "A 1907 *New York Times* Article[27] shows that meat causes cancer. A century later, many people still haven't heard the news."[28]

Heart Disease. In 2005, the China Study examined the link between meat consumption, dairy foods, and such illnesses as coronary heart disease, diabetes, breast cancer, prostate cancer, and bowel cancer. The authors concluded that people who eat a plant-based diet—a diet devoid of meats, fish, dairies, eggs, and all animal by-products—will avoid, reduce, or even reverse the development of numerous diseases.[29] A team of scientists at Loma Linda University School of Public Health in California, AgroParisTech, and the Institut National de la Recherche Agronomique in Paris, France, recently published a study concluding that eating meat is associated with a 60 percent increase in the risk of heart disease and that plant-based proteins have considerable benefit to the heart. They concluded that

> associations between the "Meat" and "Nuts & Seeds" protein factors and cardiovascular outcomes were strong and could not be ascribed to other associated nutrients considered to be important for cardiovascular health. Healthy diets

can be advocated based on protein sources, preferring low contributions of protein from meat and higher intakes of plant protein from nuts and seeds.[30]

Breast Cancer. A 2014 Harvard study found that just one serving a day of red meat during adolescence was associated with a 22 percent higher risk of pre-menopausal breast cancer, and that the same red meat consumption in adulthood was associated with an overall 13 percent higher risk of breast cancer.[31]

Obesity. Meat eaters are three times more likely to be obese than vegetarians, and nine times more likely than vegans. On average, vegans are ten to twenty pounds lighter than meat eaters. Vegan diets promote higher metabolic rates, around 16 percent faster for vegans compared with meat eaters.[32]

Life Expectancy. According to a study published in *JAMA Internal Medicine*, vegetarians may live longer than meat eaters. The study concludes, "Vegetarian diets are associated with lower all-cause mortality and with some reductions in cause-specific mortality."[33]

Sickest Population. It is interesting to note that the United States, "where meat is consumed at more than three times the global average,"[34] is one of the sickest nations in the world.

> The United States spends much more money on health care than any other country. Yet Americans die sooner and experience more illness than residents in many other countries. While the length of life has improved in the United States, other countries have gained life years even faster, and our relative standing in the world has fallen over the past half century.[35]

The rate of obesity, heart disease, high cholesterol, and diabetes in the United States has been growing exponentially.[36] Considering the deleterious health consequences caused by consumption of animal products and the benefits of a plant-based diet, it is not hard to understand why a temperate individual would avoid animals products. Besides exploiting and killing animals, which are callous practices, consuming animal products is self-destructive from a health standpoint. In terms of VE, it evinces a lack of respect for one's body and a lack of discipline over one's appetite. I believe it is reasonable to say that an individual who has the virtue of temperance will not eat animal products. Surely, one may argue that the idea of temperance is an idea of moderation, and eating animal products in moderation (perhaps) will not be as harmful. However, we have to consider three points: first, that eating animal products is not essential in any sense to human beings.[37] Second, most people in the world have access to an abundance of plant-based food. And third, eating animal products is in fact unhealthful. Consequently, meat eating is practiced out of pleasure or tradition, and therefore it is a mark of intemperance. According to VE, regarding ethical eating, the question is what a temperate agent would do in our circumstances. By "our" I refer to those who are not stranded on a desert island but have readily available plant-based food. It seems to me that, given the potential harm of an animal-based diet and its being superfluous to humans, the temperate individual will avoid it. Is it possible to be temperate by consuming animal products in moderation? I believe that due to the very fact that this type of food is intrinsically unhealthful to human beings, moderation does not apply here. It would be like taking poison in moderation—it's still poison. Considering that humans do not have any nutritional requirement to consume animal products, it is a mark of intemperance to indulge in animal products. Moreover, it does not require a tremendous sacrifice to avoid animal products and eat a plant-based diet. As Aristotle pointed out, one should not indulge in certain bodily pleasures when one can "easily accustom oneself to resist pleasures...and the modes of accustoming oneself are quite safe."[38]

At the end of Book III of the *Ethics*, concluding the discussion of what it means for a person to be temperate and intemperate, Aristotle reminds us that the appetitive element in a temperate person ought to be in harmony with reason; for the aim of both is what is noble, and the temperate person's appetite is for the right thing, in the right way, and at the right time, and this is what reason requires as well.[39] Considering the danger of consuming animal products to human health, it would seem rational to avoid animal products altogether rather than trying to salvage a type of food that is intrinsically unhealthful to our organism just for taste or tradition.

A correct analysis of temperance thus reveals that a temperate individual would embrace ethical veganism. In fact, ethical veganism argues that since killing animals for food is unnecessary and also not conducive to health, it is immoral. And since animal products are not necessary and their consumption is unhealthful, animal products are the wrong food for humans. In this sense, ethical veganism is an expression of temperance, because the temperate individual regulates his or her appetite for the right food. As illustrated above, health sciences do not speak in favor of an animal-based diet but rather confirm the benefits of a plant-based diet. In light of these facts, meat eaters who have easy access to an abundance of plant-based food of equal or superior nutritional value to animal-based food are intemperate because they unnecessarily indulge in foods that are not essential or conducive to health—and, in fact, as health sciences continue to show, animal-based food can have deleterious effects on our health.

Another virtue that can provide an ethical basis for veganism is compassion. Compassion is not one of the classical virtues proposed by Aristotle; it is, however, widely recognized as a virtue by most contemporary moral thinkers. However, Aristotle discusses how compassion is an important moral feeling that the virtuous individual possesses and uses at the right time and for the right reason. He defines compassion as follows:

> Let compassion be a sort of distress at an apparent evil, destructing or distressing, which happens to someone who doesn't deserve it, and which one might expect to happen to oneself or someone close to one and this when it appear near.[40]

For Aristotle, compassion is the pain felt at the misfortune one believes to have befallen another when the suffering is serious rather than trivial; the belief is held that the suffering is undeserved, and the sufferer may be without fault, or the deplorable consequences may outweigh the fault, affecting our sense of injustice.[41] With regard to animals, it is not hard, I argue, to imagine what a compassionate person would do. Also, I want to note that most moral thinkers agree that compassion is an important moral feeling, though they might object that unaided compassion cannot serve as a moral guide. Inasmuch as ethical veganism is concerned, animals are used as a source of food (and more) though they are not necessary. What would a compassionate person do, then? Compassion is an important moral feeling connected with a good moral character that we need to have "at the right time, about the right things, towards the right people, for the right end, and in the right way, is the mean and best; and this is the business of virtue."[42] Since virtue involves having the right feelings and performing the right action, a compassionate individual will not only feel compassion but will also act compassionately. As Roger Crisp writes,

> Someone with the virtue of compassion will act in ways characteristic of someone who feels compassion appropriately. She will offer the right kind of help in the right kind of way rather than ignoring the other's plight on the one hand, or providing the wrong sort of assistance, such as smothering the other with her concern.[43]

Indeed, the compassionate person does not just suffer on behalf of others, as it were, but is motivated to make a concerted effort to help and to alleviate the pain of others. Therefore, the idea of a compassionate individual is that he or she will perform compassionate actions in the proper way—that is, knowing what she is doing, choosing the actions appropriately for their own sake (or, for the sake of the "noble," as Aristotle puts it), given the situation at hand, and performing them from a well-grounded disposition.[44]

What are the relevant factors here? With regard to animals, what are the actions of a compassionate individual toward them? To be compassionate means to be concerned about others' pain, with the hope of alleviating it and that some positive good will emerge from the sufferer's unfortunate situation. Since being virtuous entails performing the proper action from a well-grounded disposition, it follows that being compassionate entails being altruistic—that is, acting in such a way as to help others who are suffering. A compassionate individual takes action to increase or maintain others' happiness. Since most animals are capable of living a pleasant life if respected, but a horrible one if exploited, a compassionate individual would avoid practices that cause pain to animals and also would try to maintain their happiness. Notice that this view is compatible with the thesis that animal suffering is qualitatively different from human suffering. I am not arguing that animal suffering and enjoyment and human suffering and enjoyment are qualitatively the same. My claim is that killing an animal just for the sake of eating steak or eggs, for example, is callous when equally or better nutritious plant-based alternatives are readily available.

A compassionate individual has empathy. Empathy "recognizes connection with an understanding of the circumstances of the other."[45] An empathetic individual tries to understand thoroughly the situation and circumstances of others and cares about their well-being. These "others" may be close to us or far away, other humans or non-human animals. For example, empathy enables us to extend our love to victims of some natural catastrophe who may live on the other side of the world. In the case of our treatment of non-human animals, the compassionate individual has empathy for them and tries to understand what matters for them. A compassionate individual, therefore, will not merely try to alleviate the pain of an animal who is about to be slaughtered by caressing him or by giving him a tranquillizer or by making his death as quick as possible. This would not be the full expression of compassion. Rather, a compassionate individual who has empathy also recognizes that animals not only wish to avoid pain, but also wish to survive and flourish. Consequently, by definition, a compassionate person would oppose all forms of animal exploitation. But just like other virtues, compassion seems to lie between two excesses. One way, for example, an individual could be too compassionate is by putting his own well-being at risk. It would be a form of excess compassion if one refused to wash his hands to protect germs, or if he denied food to his children to feed strangers, or if he allowed rats to take over his apartment. Conversely, one would not be compassionate enough if he deliberately killed animals for fun or just for the sake of it, or, in the instant case, if he had an abundance of nutritious plant-based food yet indulged in eating products derived from the exploitation and death of animals. Ethical veganism is the idea that we should avoid using animals for food or clothing when we have equal or superior readily available plant-based alternatives, as is the case in many developed countries.

A typical objection is that eating meat would seem consistent with compassion as long as animals are treated with respect. However, from my evaluation of compassion, it does not appear to be the case. Many people may claim that the compassionate way to use animals for food is to allow them to live a happy life. This attitude, however, evinces a failure to be compassionate or an incompleteness of the virtue of compassion. For VE, it is not sufficient to be compassionate only in some instances.[46] The very idea of compassion is not only to suffer with or share others' suffering but also to make a positive contribution to their happiness. If we truly treat animals well and are concerned about their well-being, it seems peculiar that we might do this with the intention of eventually killing them to have them as food. Using the adverb "compassionately" to modify the verb "kill" is not sufficient to make killing a compassionate act. Therefore, one may not claim to be compassionate in the complete sense of the virtue if one's actions involve acts such as killing animals merely because their cooked flesh tastes good and gives them a great deal of pleasure. One must be thoroughly and consistently compassionate toward animals. Also, one is not truly compassionate by simply refraining from directly being cruel to or directly exploiting animals. One must also not be party to the exploitation of animals; one must not purchase leather, fur, or meat, or choose to remain ignorant or inactive by shrugging it off and saying that he cannot do anything about it. Here I consider as a premise that for virtually all people who live in affluent societies, eating meat is a caprice rather than a strict necessity. Consequently, it is in no way compassionate to kill an animal for food, for entertainment, or for fun, or even if it is done in a way that minimizes or avoids pain. As Stephens points out, a "compassionate person would feel moral discomfort, or even revulsion, enjoying something made possible only by the suffering of another."[47] Therefore, insofar as veganism is the position according to which we should not kill animals or use their body parts and by-products when other equal or superior plant-based foods or clothing are readily available, veganism is an expression of virtue—more precisely, it is an expression of compassion.

Another aspect of virtue that enables us to see what is virtuous about veganism is what Aristotle calls the crown of the virtues—that is, greatness of the soul—which he discusses in the *Ethics*, Book IV.3. Greatness of the soul consists in thinking oneself worthy of great things and being concerned about honor. A great-souled individual, in other words, possesses great moral qualities, such as compassion, temperance, and a sense of justice in the sense of what is right or wrong in a given circumstance. What emerges from an analysis of what it is to be a great-souled individual is "the sort of person to do good," and "it would be quite unfitting [for a great-souled individual] to run away with his arms swinging, or to commit an injustice."[48] The kind of picture we get of the great-souled individual is a magnanimous and just individual who cares about others and is not afraid to help the vulnerable.

A great-souled individual must be just. Being just means avoiding actions in accordance with vice, such as committing adultery or wanton violence.[49] The just individual is a fair individual.[50] One might object that Aristotle is talking here about civic justice. But I believe his definition of the just in terms of a fair individual is broad enough to be relevant to the question of our treatment of animals. Aristotle views the just and fair individual as a great-souled individual. He says "the best is . . . the one who exercises [his virtue] in relation to others" and what "tends to produce or to preserve happiness."[51] In other words, the virtuous individual, as a great-souled individual, would be against wanton violence, exploiting people or animals. A fair individual recognizes that hurting animals intentionally is unfair. Also, a fair-minded individual acts out of justice to ensure that everyone receives what he or she deserves. Being fair means ensuring that others receive the deserved treatment. For example, it is unfair to deny certain benefits to a group of people solely on the basis of, say, their color, gender, or race. The fair individual is fair to all, regardless of their skin color, nationality, height, age, species, and so on. Also, it seems plausible to say that, following this idea of fairness, it is unfair to raise and kill animals for food when plant-based foods are readily available. Eating and using animals typically causes countless animals to suffer and be killed for trivial reasons, such as taste, fashion, and amusement. In societies where plant food is readily available and abundant, using animals as a source of food is, by definition, unfair. Virtue ethics here agrees with deontology and consequentialism about the moral importance of taking into account animals' conscious experience and their capacity to suffer; but while utilitarianism argues that these two factors should be taken into account so as to maximize overall happiness or preference, and deontology regards them as the basis for duty or rights, for VE animals' mental capacity and their capacity to feel pain or pleasure inform our virtuous character of their moral importance. That is to say, animals' conscious experience and their capacity to have a great life, or a miserable one, give us an objective reason to be compassionate toward them and to treat them with respect.

The notion that animals are conscious and feel pain is no longer a controversial one. For example, studies now show that in addition to large animals, "there is adequate behavioral and physiological evidence to support pain attributions to fish."[52] As cognitive ethologist Donald Griffin points out, it is arbitrary to deny animals a level of self-awareness; most of the animals that are typically regarded as food—cows, pigs, lambs, chickens, and others—are conscious and aware of their own bodies and actions. Animal thoughts and emotions may be simple compared to humans' in the sense that perhaps animals can think only of matters of immediate importance; in this sense, their awareness of the world is said to be not as sophisticated as that of human beings. However, Griffin argues, consciousness is not an all-or-nothing attribute. Most animals are complex enough to be able to organize and retain information about many aspects of their lives. For example, they recognize different odors to which they react in different ways, suggesting many subjective feelings and awareness.[53] If this is correct, killing such animals merely to satisfy our taste for a certain dish is immoral because they experience the world, and killing them deprives them of their future existence and experiences. When we consider carefully the mental capacity of animals and we consider what it is to be a great-souled individual—that is, a compassionate, magnanimous, caring, and fair individual—it seems quite unlikely to claim that a great-souled individual might treat animals with compassion (for instance in very high welfare production systems) and then decide to eventually kill them with minimal pain and suffering in order to eat them. The practice of killing animals to eat them—not out of necessity but rather for trivial reasons—is not in accordance with the actions of a great-souled individual who is compassionate, temperate, and fair. Again, considering that eating meat is not required to thrive, and considering that in well-developed societies there is an abundance of plant-based food of equal or superior nutritional value to meat, it follows that killing animals and eating them is immoral. If it is not out of necessity, then eating meat is a practice justified merely by tradition, taste, convenience, or other trivial reasons. Animals experience the world. They are individuals. Although they may not be, cognitively speaking, as sophisticated as human beings, it would seem that they want to enjoy their existence. It follows that tradition, convenience, and taste are not good reasons to use animals, even "humanely." If we are consistently fair, we will not merely try to ameliorate the living conditions of animals with the intent to eventually turn them into food or clothes, or try to kill them with minimal pain. Rather, if we are fair, compassionate, and temperate, we will avoid exploiting them in the first place. Using their bodies, their skin, their milk, their fur, or their eggs is therefore immoral as well. Ethical veganism argues that when plant food is readily available, using animals for food is unnecessary, unfair, cruel, and also unhealthful, and thus it is an immoral practice. Therefore, ethical veganism embodies the virtues of compassion, fairness, temperance, and what it is to be a great-souled person.

EATING MEAT AND THE DESTRUCTION OF THE ENVIRONMENT

A further way to show that using animals for food is callous, intemperate, unfair, and unhealthful, and that acquiring the virtues leads to ethical veganism is that raising animals for food can be harmful to the environment and, in turn, can be harmful to humans. Meat consumption takes a serious toll on the environment. According to the Environmental Working Group, the production, processing, and distribution of meat requires excessive amounts of pesticide, fertilizer, fuel, feed, and water. As a result, toxic chemicals are released into the air and water.[54] Studies consistently indicate that plant-based diets have the largest environmental benefits compared to meat-based diets.[55] Conversely, meat-based diets are damaging for the environment. Raising animals for food requires massive amounts of land, food, water, and energy. It is a known fact that a staggering amount of global greenhouse-gas emission is caused by animal agriculture.[56] What's more, unfortunately, the amount of food required to feed livestock could feed more people. According to ecologist David Pimentel of Cornell University's College of Agriculture and Life Sciences, "If all the grain currently fed to livestock in the United States were consumed directly by people, the number of people who could be fed would be nearly 800 million."[57]

Considering that animal products contribute negatively to the degradation of the environment, ethical veganism is an important step toward a better future. According to the United Nations, a global move toward a diet devoid of animal products is necessary to "save the world from the worst impacts of climate change."[58] Growing crops to feed animals, cleaning pollution from factory farms, and satisfying animals' thirst requires an enormous amount of water. The numbers among studies vary, but to get an idea, consider that a single cow can drink up to fifty gallons of water per day, and double that amount in hot weather.[59] And according to the USGS Water Science School, "about 460 gallons for 1/4 lb. of beef, or about 1750 L per 113 g" of water is required.[60]

Considering the great number of animals raised for food, it is not surprising that they produce enormous amounts of waste that inevitably pollute our waterways more than all other industrial sources combined. Also, pesticides, chemicals, fertilizers, hormones, and antibiotics involved in animal agriculture degrade the environment and cause human health problems. Runoff from factory farms and livestock grazing pollutes our rivers and lakes. The USEPA notes that bacteria and viruses are carried by the runoff and contaminate groundwater.[61]

Furthermore, using land to grow crops to feed animals is inefficient. According to the UN Convention to Combat Desertification,

> In India, annual grain consumption per person amounts to around 400 lb. per year, while in the United States, it is 1500 lb. It is crucial to understand that of these 1500 lb., only 300 lb. are directly consumed as bread, cereals or pastry. The great bulk of the rest is used for meat production. While three pounds of grain are needed to produce a one-pound gain in live weight of pigs, seven pounds are needed for a one-pound gain of a cow's live weight.[62]

It takes almost twenty times less land to feed someone on a plant-based (vegan) diet than it does to feed a meat eater since the crops are consumed directly instead of being used to feed animals.

CONCLUSION

I have argued that a virtue-based approach is the correct moral framework to justify ethical veganism. I pointed out that deontic and consequentialist accounts are incapable of defending the conclusion that we should be or become vegans. Essentially, the reason these moral approaches fail is that they lose sight of the important issue about our treatment of animals by focusing on abstract principles such as duty or rights or maximization of utility; they also try, unpersuasively, to show a symmetry between the moral value of humans and that of animals. My focus has been to show that it is more plausible to frame a defense of ethical veganism by starting from a question of what it is to be what Aristotle calls a great-souled individual. As I have argued, this individual is compassionate, just, and temperate. Consequently, acquiring these virtues and acting from them will motivate ethical veganism. That is to say, a virtuous individual is compassionate, caring, and sensitive to cruelty and unfairness to animals, and therefore these moral qualities will lead to ethical veganism.

NOTES

1. This revival began with the famous G. E. M. Anscombe's article "Modern Moral Philosophy," *Philosophy* 33, no. 124 (1958).
2. Hursthouse, *On Virtue Ethics*, 3.
3. PETA, "Is It OK to Eat Eggs from Chickens I've Raised in My Backyard?" http://www.peta.org/about-peta/faq/is-it-ok-to-eat-eggs-from-chickens-ive-raised-in-my-backyard/.
4. Vegan Society, "We've Come a Long Way!" (2016), https://www.vegansociety.com/about-us/history.
5. "What Is Veganism," https://www.thoughtco.com/what-is-veganism-127598.
6. Aristotle, *Nichomachean Ethics* IV. 3.
7. See the case of Singer's mother discussed in chapter 2.
8. Donovan, "Feminism," 306.
9. BBC News, "Fraudster Bernard Madoff and Wife 'Attempted Suicide,'" October 26, 2011. Retrieved October 27, 2011, https://www.bbc.come/news/business-14336043.
10. "Bernie Madoff's Son Mark Commits Suicide," https://nypost.com/2010/12/11/bernie-madoffs-son-mark-commits-suicide/.
11. Bob Breindenbach, "Homeless Man Who Admitted to 23-Year-Old Unsolved Murder Gets 30 Years in Prison," *Providence Journal*, http://www.providencejournal.com/article/20150818/news/150819346.
12. Plato, *Republic*, IV.445a–b.
13. Aristotle, *Nichomachean Ethics*, 1106a16–25.
14. Ibid., 1098a12–18.
15. Ibid., 1106b36–1107a2.
16. Ibid., 1104a12–13.
17. Ibid., 1106a29–b8.
18. Ibid., 1118a, 10.
19. Ibid., 1128a, 25.
20. Ibid., 1118a, 15.
21. Ibid., 1119a, 15.
22. See P. J. Tuso, M. H. Ismail, B.P. Ha, and C. Bartolotto, "Nutritional Update for Physicians: Plant-Based Diets," *The Permanente Journal* 17, no. 2 (2013): 61–66, doi: https://doi.org/10.7812/TPP/12–085. "Research shows that plant-based diets are cost-effective, low-risk interventions that may lower body mass index, blood pressure, HbA1C, and cholesterol levels. They may also reduce the number of medications needed to treat chronic diseases and lower ischemic heart disease mortality rates. Physicians should consider recommending a plant-based diet to all their patients, especially those with high blood pressure, diabetes, cardiovascular disease, or obesity."

23. W. J. Craig, A. R. Mangels, "Position of the American Dietetic Association: Vegetarian Diets," *Am. Diet. Assoc.* 109, no. 7 (July 2009): 1266–82.

24. Midgley, 8.

25. Véronique Bouvard et al., "Carcinogenicity of Consumption of Red and Processed Meat," *The Lancet Oncology* 16, no. 16 (2015): 1599–1600.

26. Cancer Council NSW, "Meat and Cancer," https://www.cancercouncil.com.au/21639/cancer-prevention/diet-exercise/nutrition-diet/fruit-vegetables/meat-and-cancer/#ScVzbuPsBRpqsQZg.99.

27. "Cancer Increasing among Meat Eaters," *New York Times*, September 24, 1907, https://timesmachine.nytimes.com/timesmachine/1907/09/24/101857679.pdf.

28. http://www.pcrm.org/nbBlog/index.php/1907-new-york-times-article-shows-that-meat-causes-cancer-a-century-later-many.

29. Colin T. Campbell, *The China Study: The Most Comprehensive Study of Nutrition Ever Conducted and the Startling Implications for Diet, Weight Loss, and Long-Term Health* (Dallas, TX: BenBella Books, 2006).

30. Marion Tharrey et al., "Patterns of Plant and Animal Protein Intake Are Strongly Associated with Cardiovascular Mortality: The Adventist Health Study-2 Cohort," https://doi.org/10.1093/ije/dyy030.

31. Amy Roder, "Red Meat Consumption and Breast Cancer Risk," October 9, 2014, https://www.hsph.harvard.edu/news/features/red-meat-consumption-and-breast-cancer-risk/.

32. T. Montalcini et al., "High Vegetable Fats Intake Is Associated with High Resting Energy Expenditure in Vegetarians," *Nutrients* 7, no. 7 (2015): 5933–5947. G. Fraser and E. Haddad, "Hot Topic: Vegetarianism, Mortality and Metabolic Risk: The New Adventist Health Study." Report presented at Academy of Nutrition and Dietetic (Food and Nutrition Conference) Annual Meeting, October 7, 2012, Philadelphia, PA.

33. "Vegetarian Dietary Patterns and Mortality in Adventist Health Study 2," *JAMA Intern Med.* 173, no. 13 (2013): 1230–1238, doi:https://doi.org/10.1001/jamainternmed.2013.6473.

34. "Trends in Meat Consumption in the United States," *Public Health Nutr.* 14, no. 4 (April 2011): 575–583. doi:https://doi.org/10.1017/S1368980010002077; "Kings of the Carnivores: Who Eats Most Meat?" *The Economist*, April 30, 2012, https://www.economist.com/graphic-detail/2012/04/30/kings-of-the-carnivores.

35. Institute of Medicine and National Research Council, *U.S. Health in International Perspective: Shorter Lives, Poorer Health* (Washington, DC: National Academies Press, 2013).

36. Institute of Medicine and National Research Council, *U.S. Health in International Perspective*.

37. See W. J. Craig and A. R. Mangels, "Position of the American Dietetic Association: Vegetarian Diets," *Am. Diet. Assoc.* 109, no. 7 (July 2009): 1266–1282.

38. Aristotle, *Nichomachean Ethics* 1119a.25.

39. Ibid., 1119b.15.

40. Aristotle, *Ars Rhetorica*, ed. W. D. Ross (Oxford: Clarendon Press, 1959), 2.8, 1385b 13–16.

41. Ibid., 1386a6–7, 1385b14, b34–1386a1, 1386b7, b10, b12, b13, 1386b14–15; and Aristotle, *De Arte Poetica*, ed. R. Kassel (Oxford: Clarendon Press, 1965), 1453a4, 5.

42. Aristotle, *Nichomachean Ethics* II.6, 1106b18–19, 1106b21–7.

43. Roger Crisp, "Compassion and Beyond," *Ethical Theory and Moral Practice* 11, no. 3, Papers Presented at the Annual Conference of the British Society for Ethical Theory, Bristol, July 2007, 243.

44. Aristotle, *Nichomachean Ethics* II.4, 1105a.

45. Lori Gruen, *Entangled Empathy: An Alternative Ethic for Our Relationship with Animals* (New York: Lantern Books, 2014) 45.

46. See Hursthouse, *On Virtue Ethics*, 14.

47. William O. Stephens, "Five Arguments for Vegetarianism," *Philosophy in the Contemporary World* 1, no. 4 (1994): 25–39, 33.

48. Aristotle, *Nichomachean Ethics* IV.3, 1123b, 30, 1124b, 18.

49. Ibid., V. 1129b, 21.

50. Ibid., 1129b.

51. Ibid., 1129b, 18.
52. Colin Allen, "Animal Pain," *Nous* 38, no. 4 (2004): 617–643.
53. See Donald R. Griffin, *Animal Minds Beyond: Cognition to Consciousness* (Chicago: University of Chicago Press, 2001).
54. Environmental Working Group, "Meat Eater's Guide" (2008), https://www.ewg.org/meateatersguide/interactive-graphic/meat-consumption/.
55. L. Aleksandrowicz et al., "The Impacts of Dietary Change on Greenhouse Gas Emissions, Land Use, Water Use, and Health: A Systematic Review," *PLoS ONE* 11, no. 11: e0165797, https://doi.org/10.1371/journal.pone.0165797.
56. Rachel Premack, "Meat Is Horrible," *Washington Post*, July 3, 2016, https://www.washingtonpost.com/news/wonk/wp/2016/06/30/how-meat-is-destroying-the-planet-in-seven-charts/?utm_term=.fa399b2b7544.
57. "How Does Meat in the Diet Take an Environmental Toll?" *Scientific American*, https://www.scientificamerican.com/article/meat-and-environment/.
58. UNEP, "Assessing the Environmental Impact of Consumption and Production," a Report of the Working Group on the Environmental Impacts of Products and Materials to the International Panel for Sustainable Resource Management (2010).
59. Institute of Agriculture and Natural Resources Producer Question from 2016 Q. How much water do cows drink per day? (July 19, 2016).
60. USGS, "The Water Content of Things: How Much Water Does It Take to Grow a Hamburger?" https://water.usgs.gov/edu/activity-watercontent.php.
61. The U.S. Environmental Protection Agency, "National Enforcement Initiative: Preventing Animal Waste from Contaminating Surface and Ground Water," https://www.epa.gov/enforcement/national-enforcement-initiative-preventing-animal-waste-contaminating-surface-and-ground.
62. UN Convention to Combat Desertification, "New ISO Standard to Combat Land Degradation," June 11, 2017.

Chapter Seven

Some Objections

BEING VEGAN IS NOT FOR EVERYONE

Is my argument applicable only to those of us who have the fortune to live in affluent societies that enjoy an abundance of plant-based food and alternatives to wool, leather, and other animal-based by-products? Such circumstances, I believe, demand compassion, temperance, fairness, and magnanimity in our relationship with animals. But does this mean that people who live in non-affluent societies are morally justified in eating and using animals? I do endorse the view that there are absolute rights and wrongs. I believe, for example, that murder, adultery, child abuse, slavery, and more are objectively wrong. That is, there are no circumstances in which they could possibly be right. Also, I believe that the act of killing animals or humans is disgraceful and inherently wrong. Granted, there are circumstances that justify killing humans or animals. But it is not as if the justifications, whatever they might be, magically turn a disgraceful event, such as killing, into a good one. The main characteristic of the virtuous person is that she does the best thing in a situation, all things considered. There are possible circumstances in which a virtuous character is compatible with using animals. Such circumstances might involve, for example, a population that has no other source of sustenance but animals, or a lifeboat hypothetical—that is, a situation in which a person or a group of people are stranded on a desert island with no food other than animals.

These, however, are exceptions that must be evaluated to see how they affect ethical veganism. In the case of being stranded on a desert island, is it obvious that one would be morally justified in eating animals? That obviously depends on many factors: Are there plants available on this hypothetical island? Or are the conditions on the island hostile to plants? If plants cannot grow at all, how could animals even exist on such an island? But let us assume that one is stranded on an island that has a very hostile environment and neither plants nor animals exist. Suppose one finds a large reserve ration consisting of canned meat and cheese. That's the only food. Should one eat the meat and cheese and survive or be vegan and die? Even if one decided to eat the meat to survive, this is an isolated disgrace that does not undermine the morality of avoiding animal-based food. Ethical veganism would still be a way of life conducive to the flourishing of humans. In such a case, then, it would be hard or impossible to flourish. Luck, and our living conditions, no doubt, can affect a good life.

With regard to other circumstances, I acknowledge that not all humans in the world *at the moment* can embrace ethical veganism. There might be small tribes of people whose religious beliefs involve eating animals. It seems unlikely that I could convince them to become vegans. But what about people whose food supplies are just scarce. Should they be vegans? Perhaps an important implication of a VE-oriented animal ethics is that affluent societies should help less-developed countries maintain plant-based diets. When people around the world experience famine, they often receive help in the way of food supplies from more fortunate countries. Thus, it seems to me that rather than sending over animal products, the more fortunate countries should help the less fortunate by sending plant-based food. In fact, in the United States, the Defense Logistics Agency developed Humanitarian Daily Rations (HDRs) to feed large populations of displaced people or refugees under emergency conditions. These daily rations provide optimal nutrition and calories for individuals and are devoid of animal products or by-products.

Furthermore, consider that some populations do have plant food in abundance but do not use it. As Richard Oppenlander notes in *Food Choice and Sustainability*, for example,

> In Ethiopia, over 40 percent of the population is considered hungry or starving, yet the country has 50 million cattle (one of the largest herds in the world), as well as almost 50 million sheep and goats, and 35 million chickens, unnecessarily consuming the food, land and water... Much of their resource use must be focused on these cattle. Instead of using their food, water, topsoil, and massive amounts of land and energy to raise livestock, Ethiopia, for instance, could grow teff, an ancient and quite nutritious grain grown in that country for the past 20,000 to 30,000 years. Teff...is high in protein, with an excellent amino acid profile, is high in fiber and calcium (1 cup of teff provides more calcium than a cup of milk), and is a rich source of boron, copper, phosphorus, zinc, and iron. Seventy percent of all Ethiopia's cattle are raised pastorally in the highlands of their country, where less than 100 pounds of meat and a few gallons of milk are produced per acre of land used. Researchers have found that teff can be grown in those same areas by the same farmers at a yield of 2,000 to 3,000 pounds per acre, with more sustainable growing techniques

employed and no water irrigation—teff has been shown to grow well in water-stressed areas and it is pest resistant.[1]

There are other regions of the world where inhabitants were believed to depend on animal-based food. But in reality they can import food staples, thus avoid relying on animals for food. An example often used is the Inuit, who inhabit the artic regions of Alaska, Canada, and Greenland. Not having fields suitable to grow food for all their meals, the Inuit traditionally ate only fish and seal meat. But nowadays, the Inuit live in communities with stores, schools, and modern buildings. Modern Inuit import food grown elsewhere and buy it in local stores. In fact, according to the Inuit Cultural Online Resource, "Expensive food [is] bought at the local Co-op or Northern store, or shipped up from the south."[2]

Thus the idea is that ethical veganism is the embodiment of a virtuous life. We should be or become ethical vegans because it is important that we acquire virtues in order to live well, and the acquisition of virtues naturally makes us embrace ethical veganism. Also, according to VE, because the virtuous person is compassionate, just, temperate, and magnanimous, he or she is motivated to help others maintain their happiness and well-being or, in times of difficulty, help restore their happiness. Thus the reasons people in affluent societies eat meat and animal products is typically lack of virtue, such as those discussed earlier. And the reason less-fortunate people eat meat and animal products is not necessarily that they don't have access to plant-based food. It is a more complicated matter than that. It is often, once again, due to lack of virtue. Consuming meat and animal products is a normal practice for many people. But what is normal is often not moral. Dietary habits, like many other aspects of life, traditions, beliefs, and customs, are normally embraced or not embraced. People eat meat because, like many other things, eating meat is a practice passed down from generations. But what is the moral justification for doing it? One of the most impressive notions in philosophy, and especially in moral philosophy, is that in any field of study, it is possible to find strong arguments from opposite sides of the spectrum. There is a solid literature in support of dualism, for example, and there is a solid literature in support of materialism. There is literature in favor of abortion and literature against it. However, a remarkable aspect of animal ethics is that no good arguments exist in support of eating meat. Some of the arguments I have come across are very simplistic. I shall give a few examples and discuss their plausibility.

WHERE DO WE DRAW THE LINE?

A typical response to ethical veganism is "But where do we draw the line?" Veganism, as I have defined it, is the idea that eating animals and animal products evinces a lack of essential virtues, such as temperance, compassion, fairness, and magnanimity. But to which animals am I referring? All animals? Insects too? Where do we draw the line of respect for animals? I want to say the following in regard to these questions. In general, ethical vegans should not necessarily worry about lions and zebras and perhaps liminal animals. In most cases, people do not eat lions, zebras, squirrels, or rats. In any event, the same principles should apply to all animals—that is, our attitude toward them should be guided by the virtues. Consider wild animals as an example. Why should a virtuous person's attitude be any different toward wild animals? Indeed, the virtuous person should respect them, not kill them or exploit them, and if necessary and possible, we should help them.

Regarding shellfish, one may wonder about the exact position of ethical veganism with respect to oysters, clams, and mussels. Is it moral to eat them? Most of these living beings don't have a central nervous system, and thus do not experience pain. They do have nerves, and that's enough to deter many. According to Jane A. Smith, "Most, if not all, invertebrates have the capacity to detect and respond to noxious or aversive stimuli. That is, like vertebrates, they are capable of 'nociception.'"[3] Nociception is the sensory response of the nervous system to certain harm or potential. Others may dispute this claim. Peter Singer, for example, stated that he has

> gone back and forth on this over the years. Perhaps there is a scintilla more doubt about whether oysters can feel pain than there is about plants, but I'd see it as extremely improbable. So while you could give them the benefit of the doubt, you could also say that unless some new evidence of a capacity for pain emerges, the doubt is so slight that there is no good reason for avoiding eating sustainably produced oysters.[4]

Thus, assuming that there is no issue of over-harvesting oceans or sustainability, this brings us to the original question, "Where do we draw the line?" I want to remind the reader, however, that my argument is not based on sentience and avoidance of suffering. As I stated earlier, whether a being is sentient and the amount of pain that it can experience are important factors in morality. However, VE suggests a further factor, that of moral character. This point is quite hard to argue, I admit. But the point is to focus on whether or not the act of eating mollusks is in accordance with the virtues. In my view it isn't. Shellfish feed on the dead skin of dead animals, as well as parasites. For this reason they are referred to as bottom feeders; consequently they can be a host to parasites and other harmful organisms. Most shellfish don't have a proper digestive system that filters out toxins and parasites, and consequently anything harmful absorbed into the shellfish stays in the shellfish. Due to their simple digestive system, it is difficult for them to expel waste, which is often ingested along with the shellfish. Granted, one may argue that this is not a problem if the mollusk is properly cleaned. But consider that shellfish is a living organism and, in most cases, before eating, one has to literally clean out its excrement. Obviously, this does not seem to be an issue since many people consume shellfish. But it seems to me that a food conducive to health should not be something that contains potential harmful bacteria, excrement, veins, organs, etc. Moreover, almost every type of shellfish contains contaminants, particularly mercury, and other types of heavy metals, which can lead to serious health problems.[5]

And considering that plants provide optimal nutrition for humans and improve health, I believe that the virtuous person would rationally avoid shellfish and stick to eating plants.

PLANTS SUFFER TOO

This last consideration obviously prompts the question of a moral justification for eating plants. Granted, plants are living organisms. A compassionate individual, then, must make a choice between eating animal products and eating plants. The compassionate approach is to choose to use those organisms that are less likely to be morally disrespected. For plants, "being alive" is different than it is for animals, in a way that makes it difficult to see in what sense it could be said that we wrong or disrespect a plant by eating it. Rice, mangoes, beans, bananas, lettuce, or broccoli do not seem to have conscious experiences or to be concerned about their existence. It is very unlikely that they enjoy life and the company of their parents and friends, like animals and people do. Furthermore, the most important aspect of VE as it relates to the question of whether plants can feel pain and whether veganism is a compassionate moral position is this: VE concerns organisms that are alive, but it also concerns nature. It is not the case that a virtuous individual would have no moral feelings or respect for mountains and water, but only for living and breathing organisms. This is a mistaken conception of VE. As Murdoch argues, "The moral life...is something that goes on continually, not something that switches off in between the occurrence of explicit moral choices. What happens in between such choices is indeed what is crucial."[6] The virtuous individual is respectful of all things—mountains, rivers, and the whole of nature. His eating choices are informed by virtue, and his actions are always appropriate in relation to the good of not only himself, but also nature as a whole. Therefore, vegans eat plants because it is consistent with temperance, compassion, magnanimity, and fairness to do so. It is, most importantly, as I hope to have shown, reasonable to believe that a great-souled individual eats a simple diet of vegetables and avoids food that is not essential and can be harmful, such as animal-based food. Furthermore, the attitude of a virtuous person is such that he or she respects all nature and takes heed not to damage or destroy it, recognizing that human beings are just a part of nature, which is essential to their flourishing.

Therefore, it would be contrary to virtue, for example, to deliberately damage or destroy plants. But the fact is that plants provide a vast variety of fruits that can be eaten without being imprisoned or tortured, disrespected, killed, or separated from family and friends. In a metaphorical sense, plants want us to eat their fruit so that their genes can propagate. These considerations make us realize that there are degrees of moral responses toward different forms of life. The degree of compassion, temperance, fairness, and magnanimity that we have for a cow need not be the same as that for a mango. Therefore, a virtuous individual avoids using animal products because their consumption is shown to be unhealthful, exploiting animals causes them unnecessary suffering, and it contributes to the degradation of the environment; all these issues are easily avoided by using plant food and plant-based by-products.[7] It seems to me to follow that the virtuous person also avoids wearing leather and using animal by-products since these are not essential to flourishing. In other words, using animals for food disrespects animals, moreover it disrespects our moral integrity. Animal by-products are typically obtained through practices that make animals suffer or that disrespect them. It is interesting to note that in addition to causing unnecessary suffering to the animals, using animals for food also causes unnecessary psychological suffering to those individuals who care for animals and wish they were left alone.[8] But in the case of plants, although they are living organisms, our using them does not require the same cruel practices that inflict pain upon animals.

These questions about drawing lines seem to me to make sense in a context of an ethic that emphasizes universal rules or one that proposes a common denominator for respecting animals—such as sentience—as the locus of morality. The point of VE is not to draw lines, because, as I have explained, VE is a moral approach that deemphasizes universal rules and consequences and focuses instead on the character of the agent. An agent who has a consistently benevolent, compassionate, temperate, and just character will always behave in ways that are benevolent, compassionate, temperate, and just. He will always act well. Conversely, an agent who is not virtuous will have to rely upon and follow universal rules or prescriptions derived from some utilitarian calculus; but there is no guarantee that the agent will be willing to act according to those rules or that the agent will be satisfied by his required actions. When we approach morality from virtue, we are asked to take into account the relevant facts of a given situation rather than abstracting those facts. In other words, a utilitarian, for example, may propose that in our dealings with animals we give equal consideration to all those beings that have preferences. The utilitarian, then, may draw a line and declare, for example, that because a fetus or a mosquito is not the kind of being whose preferences could be satisfied, we cast them outside the moral community. Kantian ethics, as illustrated in chapter 1, is another perfect example of this. According to Kant, the so-called line has to be drawn in accordance with rationality; and since animals are not rational, we have no direct moral duty to them.

VE sees the issue differently. A compassionate individual, for example, is concerned about the well-being of all living things. He respects all creatures because all have dignity and deserve moral respect. For a virtuous individual, it is not the case that only certain beings have moral worth while others are absolutely worthless or irrelevant. This is an attitude embedded in the virtues. A virtuous individual respects insects in that he does not kill them intentionally or take pleasure in torturing or killing them. Since he also respects nature, he will not destroy plants or pollute waters. At the same time, VE is consistent in its approach because it does not categorically prohibit killing animals who threaten our lives or insects that, for example, might infest our homes. In such circumstances, a virtuous individual is morally consistent. With regard to ethical veganism, considering that we can conduct our lives without using animals for food, clothing, or other purposes, exploiting animals is inconsistent with the virtues.

EATING MEAT IS AN ENJOYABLE EXPERIENCE

Some argue that they really enjoy eating meat. The pleasure derived from eating animals and animal-based foods is important—to meat eaters. But how important? First, I often wonder whether people really enjoy eating meat and to what extent. I am convinced that not too many people would really eat a slab of animal flesh unless it has been coated in spices and sauces and then cooked. What people really like when they eat a piece of animal flesh is the final processed and cooked product. Most people are repulsed by the very idea of killing an animal. But they are even more repulsed by the sight of blood, guts, and fluids oozing out of an animal carcass. This may sound like a fallacious appeal to emotion. But I don't think that using such an appeal is inherently fallacious. Here again, I rely on Midgley's notion of the "yuck factor." Midgley rightly emphasizes the importance of listening to our deepest feelings to inform our moral evaluation of issues:

> Feeling is an essential part of our moral life, though of course not the whole of it. Heart and mind are not enemies or alternative tools. They are complementary aspects of a single process. Whenever we seriously judge something to be wrong, strong feeling necessarily accompanies the judgment. Someone who does not have such feelings—someone who has merely a theoretical interest in morals, who doesn't feel any indignation or disgust and outrage about things like slavery and torture—has missed the point of morals altogether.[9]

Midgley's approach involves acknowledgment of our deep emotions regarding an act (heart) and rational calculations (head). Rational calculation is often important, but to discount the heart's yuck factor forthright is to limit our moral understanding. The yuck factor is the reaction of inarticulate moral intuition that must be seriously considered because it requires time to rise to the rational level and be articulated.

> Feelings always incorporate thoughts—often ones that are not yet fully articulated—and reasons are always found in response to particular sorts of feelings. On both sides, we need to look for the hidden partners. We have to articulate the thoughts that underlie emotional objections and also note the emotional element in contentions that may claim to be purely rational. The best way to do this is often to start by taking the intrinsic objections more seriously. If we look below the surface of what seems to be mere feeling we may find thoughts that show how the two aspects are connected.[10]

Therefore, I believe that the nearly uniform aversion of people to blood, bodily fluid, bad odor, and other "yucky" aspects involved in meat production, far from being a mere subjective factor, shows that there is something intrinsically wrong about it. Not surprisingly, the yucky aspects of meat production are hidden from plain sight. And not surprisingly, meat eaters typically consume cooked and seasoned, rather than raw, animal flesh.

People also believe that they have free choice and experience the world objectively, but research shows that beliefs influence perception—not to mention that beliefs in their turn are influenced by a number of factors over which we have no control. This sounds just like a phrase taken by Baron d'Holbach's writing on determinism.[11] I am not suggesting that we are determined in the way d'Holbach argued we are. My point is simply that there is a substantial amount of psychological research confirming that, specifically with regard to our understanding of animals, we are, to put it bluntly, clueless. This research shows that our beliefs influence the experience of eating. In three studies, researchers tested whether their beliefs of how animals are raised can influence their experience of eating them. Samples of meat were accompanied by respective descriptions of their origins and treatment of the animals on factory farms. Some samples were said to be the product of factory farm, while others were labeled "humane." In reality, all the meat samples were identical. Interestingly, the participants of this study experienced the samples differently: meat described as "factory farmed" was perceived as looking, smelling, and tasting less pleasant than "humane" meat. The difference was even to the degree that factory farmed meat was said to taste more salty and greasy than "humane" meat. Furthermore, the participants who were told that they were eating factory farmed meat consumed less. According to the authors of this study, "These findings demonstrate that the experience of eating is not determined solely by physical properties of stimuli—beliefs also shape experience."[12]

Furthermore, I question the moral importance of taste. We enjoy all sorts of things, but the question is whether we enjoy them because they are essential or because they are enjoyed, which brings the discussion back to the importance of a temperate character. For example, it is not surprising that we enjoy sweet food because sugar is essential. What I mean is that the human body uses sugar as fuel. But there are other things that humans enjoy that are not essential. In fact, most of them are deleterious. Many enjoy smoking, drinking alcohol, taking drugs, and so on, but not because the human body requires them. It is clear that human beings in many of their practices learn to enjoy all types of experiences, both beneficial and deleterious. The important point here is that just because one enjoys something does not make it moral. One can enjoy, for example, gratuitously lying to people, but that is obviously immoral. Eating animal products is not essential and is unhealthful; but it is one of those things that people enjoy. However, it should be considered that that enjoyment derives from the death of some animals. This argument may smack as a typical appeal to pity. Perhaps it sounds like it, but it is not. I am not simply arguing that eating meat is wrong because it causes the death of animals. I am pointing out that eating meat is not essential for human health and therefore it is done only for pleasure. But pleasure is not a moral justification for allowing the death of others.

EATING ANIMALS IS NATURAL

Another argument is that eating animals is "natural." By "natural," it is meant that human beings are somehow "designed" to eat animals, as if it were a "law of nature" or the cycle of life. The issue with this argument is that it is not crystal clear that humans are "designed" to eat meat. But even if they were, that would not prove anything. Let me illustrate that with an example. Imagine you were told the truth about yourself—that is, you are a terminator adopted by a human family. In the eponymous film starring Arnold Schwarzenegger, a terminator is a human-like machine designed to destroy Sara Connor. Now imagine you were told that you are a terminator. It would be odd if you immediately changed the purpose of your existence and embarked on the mission of killing Sara Connor. Thus, even if it turned out to be true that humans are designed to eat meat, it does not follow that they must. Also, in recent years a best-selling book was published with the title of *Born to Run*.[13] This book argues that humans are creatures designed by nature to be runners. Perhaps it is true. But it does not follow that we must be runners. We all have the freedom to choose what we want to do with our lives. Most importantly, with this freedom come moral obligations. Now here the attentive reader may have noticed that my last statement seems to contradict my earlier one about plant-based food being the optimal diet designed by nature for human beings. However, my argument is not that because fruit and vegetables are humans' natural and best food, it follows that we must be ethical vegans. Obviously, we still have choice. Rather, my point is that plant-based food is humans' natural and best food. Consuming it is conducive to health. Conversely, consuming animal products is unhealthful. Good health is necessary to flourishing. Ethical veganism recommends eating plant-based food and avoiding animal-based food. Therefore we should embrace ethical veganism because it is conducive to flourishing.

What is also suspicious about the argument from nature can be explained by this thought experiment. A friend invites you over for dinner. He promised you a succulent meat-based dinner. As you are ready to sit at the table, your friend tells you that he has roasted a whole dog—that is dinner! If you were brought up in the West, you would likely be taken aback, to say the least, by your friend's dinner choice. But now ask yourself, why is it wrong to eat a dog and right to eat a cow or a pig or a turkey? This reflection should make one pause. The fact that dog is (typically) not dinner in the West is purely accidental, a socio-geographical accident. According to Dr. Melanie Joy, a professor of psychology and sociology at the University of Massachusetts Boston, this attitude evinces hypocrisy, which is due to a concept that she calls "carnism." With the term "carnism" Dr. Joy describes a devious belief system that has convinced many people that it is perfectly acceptable to eat certain animals and immoral to eat others, despite the fact that many of these animals are anatomically very similar. Meat eaters and vegetarians who consume animal products have a psychological mechanism to explain their behavior, which Joy calls the Three N's of Justification: Normal, Natural, and Necessary. But in reality, when we think about it, eating animals is none of those N's.[14]

I concur with Joy that there is no ethical way to eat animals and animal products. Furthermore, the mechanism that she describes as "carnism" is a source of injustice in terms of race, gender, and sexuality. This point reminds us of Kant's indirect duty view toward animals (see chapter 1), where Kant argues that cruel behavior toward animals can translate into cruelty toward other beings. Kant believed that this is an amphiboly of reasoning from animals to humans. That is, he believed that people mistakenly think of animals as morally important due to certain characteristics that are similar to human characteristics. But in reality, according to Kant, this is a mistake because animals are not intrinsically valuable. They are mere objects. They are not ends in themselves, but rather means to our ends. In my view, disrespecting animals makes it easy to disrespect humans, not due to an amphiboly, but rather due to the actual moral worth of animals. In my view, and the view of others like Dr. Joy, animals do have an intrinsic moral worth. Consequently, if we oppress animals, not surprisingly, we are likely to oppress other human beings. Carol J. Adams also expresses this concern. In *The Sexual Politics of Meat,* she explains the concept of "the absent referent." According to Adams, meat conceptually represents an absence, which is the death of the animal who had to die for the meat. The absent referent thus is a mechanism that covers up the violence behind eating meat. It is a sort of cognitive dissonance that protects the meat eater's conscience, a mechanism that makes animals as if they were non-existent to the selfish desire of meat eating. The absent referent separates the meat eater from animals and animals from meat dishes.

> Male dominance and animals' oppression are linked by the way that both women and animals function as absent referents in meat eating and dairy production, and that feminist theory logically contains a vegan critique . . . just as veganism covertly challenges patriarchal society. Patriarchy is a gender system that is implicit in human/animal relationships.[15]

She also discusses how eating animals objectifies them and as a result enables a mechanism that makes oppression morally justified.

> *The Sexual Politics of Meat* shows how a process of objectification, fragmentation, and consumption enables the oppression of animals so that animals are rendered being-less through technology, language, and cultural representation. Objectification permits an oppressor to view another being as an object. Once objectified, a being can be fragmented. Once fragmented, consumption happens. The consumption of a being, and the consumption of the meaning of that being's death, so that the referent point of meat changes.[16]

ANIMALS EAT OTHER ANIMALS

Many believe that since certain animals eat other animals, it is normal or natural for us to eat animals as well. Typically this is followed by the statement that humans are carnivores. I believe that many features of humans indicate that we are plant and fruit eaters. However, carnivores do not have moral choice. They eat the flesh of other animals and could not survive on a vegetarian diet. Also, it does not seem to be a fair analogy because humans and carnivore animals obtain their food in quite different ways. Carnivores do not walk into supermarkets, buy steaks or sausages, and then season and cook them like humans do. They catch their food or eat the flesh of dead animals they find on the ground. Also, carnivores eat the whole animal, flesh, hair, eyes, blood, bones, and nerves, right there on the spot. On the other hand, people buy meat in supermarkets. The meat has been conveniently cut, cleaned, and packaged for them; it is taken home, seasoned to taste, cooked, and eaten. Therefore, although humans are animals, they are different kinds of animals in that they are capable of appreciating morality in a way that non-human animals obviously cannot, and unlike most animals, humans can survive on an exclusively plant-based diet—and in fact such a diet is healthful, while a meat-based diet isn't. What this means is that eating meat is something humans have learned to do but is not necessary.

WHAT ABOUT TRADITION?

Another argument to justify animal exploitation is that it is a human tradition. Throughout the centuries, humans have always exploited animals. But why continue a tradition if it is immoral? Think about slavery. For millennia, slavery was a legitimate practice. At one point in history, many people realized the absurdity of slavery and fought to abolish it, realizing that they had been wrong. Slavery shows that many traditions or practices in human history often are unethical. Thus, the argument that humans have always eaten meat is fallacious and historically inaccurate because it is not true that humans always have eaten meat. The important point here is this: With hindsight, we all recognize the wrong of slavery. But back in those times, many people did not see the wrong in it. Now, think about what people do to animals. How can we be sure that we are ethically warranted to use them as property, kill them, eat them, wear them, etc.? How can we be sure that we are not wrong, just like the people in the past were wrong for condoning slavery?

RELIGION ALLOWS MEAT

Another argument I have heard over the years is from religious people who maintain that eating animals is not wrong because their respective religious leaders, as well as their respective religious texts, promote the consumption of meat. Now, while it is true that certain passages in religious texts recount stories of people eating animals or of God offering animals as food or even animal sacrifice, no religion that I know of prescribes consumption of meat. To put it the other way around, no religion teaches people that a vegan diet is not proper or is irreligious.

Granted, there are many passages in religious texts that clearly acknowledge consumption of meat. However, we must consider that most religious texts were written in times prior to globalization, when supermarkets did not exist, and when people did not have much choice in the way of food and knew very little about nutrition. But the important point to me is this: It seems to me the message of various religions—with the exception of Voodoo and Satanism—is peace, compassion, and love. The message of veganism is, after all, peace, compassion, and love for all sentient creatures. Conversely, using animals for food is part of a worldview that is about pain, cruelty, and profit. Thus, it would seem to me that given these premises, and considering that nowadays we can survive well on an exclusively vegan diet, religion should have no difficulty supporting ethical veganism.

EATING MEAT IS HEALTHFUL

Another main argument is that eating animal products is essential for good health. I already addressed this question earlier. The short answer is that meat and other animal-based products are not ideal for the human body and can actually cause serious health problems. It is evident from the scientific literature and from experience that the human body functions properly on plant-based food because it is full of fiber, antioxidants, unsaturated fats, essential fatty acids, phytochemicals, and cholesterol-free protein. To be sure, most of the studies I mention here do not explicitly state, "Stay away from animal products!" Many studies may even recommend—as traditionally expected—consuming animal products due to beneficial nutrients. We have heard many times that the calcium in milk is good for the bones and the omega fatty acids in fish are beneficial to us. However, while animal products may in fact contain such beneficial nutrients, we have to consider two important factors: One is that all nutrients, amino acids, omega fatty acids, vitamins, and more are readily found in plants.[17] In some cases, as for vitamin B12, requirements are easily satisfied by supplements, which are rather inexpensive and practical. And the second factor is that while animal products may contain important nutrients, eating animal products, as I have shown earlier, is not healthful. People insist on consuming animal products despite scientific research consistently showing that people who avoided animal products were much less likely to develop serious diseases. Significant studies in England and Germany, for example, showed that those who avoided animal products were about 40 percent less likely to develop cancer compared to meat eaters.[18] The conclusion reached by many studies is consistent. Vegetables and fruit help to reduce and prevent risk of several diseases, including cancer, high blood pressure, diabetes, and more. Animal products, on the other hand, are consistently found to increase risk of such diseases. Consumption of animal fat contributes to production of hormones that promote growth of cancer cells in hormone-sensitive organs such as the breast and prostate. One of the most important nutrients is fiber. Meat is devoid of fiber, phytochemicals, and other helpful nutrients that prevent risk of developing many different kinds of cancer.

Vegetarian diets and diets rich in high-fiber plant foods such as whole grains, legumes, vegetables, and fruits offer a measure of protection.[19] Fiber in particular speeds the passage of food through the colon, thus removing carcinogens; it also changes the type of bacteria present in the intestine, and therefore reduces production of carcinogenic secondary bile acids. Plant foods are rich in antioxidants and anti-cancer compounds. Consequently, vegetarians have been found by many studies to be at the lowest risk for cancer and other health issues compared to meat eaters.[20] To step back for a moment to my observation that human beings have a food that is optimal to them and animals are not human food, it seems that the consistent scientific data regarding human nutrition corroborates such an observation.[21] Animal products, contrary to what many believe, are unhealthful for humans. Consequently, the virtuous person avoids animal-based food because it is not conducive to flourishing.

NOTES

1. Richard Oppenlander, *Food Choice and Sustainability: Why Buying Local, Eating Less Meat, and Taking Baby Steps Won't Work* (Minneapolis: Langdon Street Press, 2013), 175–178.

2. Inuit Cultural Online Resource, "Explore our Culture, Modern vs Traditional Life," https://www.icor.ottawainuitchildrens.com/explore-our-culture.

3. Jane A. Smith, "A Question of Pain in Invertebrates," *ILAR Journal* 33, no. 1–2 (1991): 25.

4. Cited in Christopher Cox, "Consider the Oyster," *Slate*, April 7, 2010, http://www.slate.com/articles/life/food/2010/04/consider_the_oyster.html.

5. Ana Luísa Maulvault, Patrícia Anacleto, Vera Barbosa, et al., "Toxic Elements and Speciation in Seafood Samples from Different Contaminated Sites in Europe," *Environmental Research* 143 (November 2015).

6. Iris Murdoch, "The Idea of Perfection," in *The Sovereignty of the Good* (London: Routledge, 1970), 8.

7. Justin Worland, "How a Vegetarian Diet Could Help Save the Planet," *Time*, March 21, 2016, http://time.com/4266874/vegetarian-diet-climate-change/.

8. Singer certainly forgot to include this kind of suffering in his calculus. But my point here is not that the suffering of people who care about animals somehow figures in a utilitarian calculus; rather, my point is that unnecessary suffering, whether physical or psychological, should be avoided because causing gratuitous suffering is callous.

9. Midgley, "Biotechnology and Monstrosity," 9.

10. Ibid., 8.

11. See Baron Paul d'Holbach, "Of the System of Man's Free Agency" from *System of Nature* (1770).

12. Eric C. Anderson and Lisa Feldman Barrett, "Affective Beliefs Influence the Experience of Eating Meat," *PLOS One*, August 24, 2016, https://doi.org/10.1371/journal.pone.0160424.

13. Christopher McDougall, *Born to Run: A Hidden Tribe, Superathletes, and the Greatest Race the World Has Never Seen* (New York: Vintage, 2011).

14. See Melany Joy, *Why We Love Dogs, Eat Pigs, and Wear Cows: An Introduction to Carnism* (Newburyport, MA: Conari Press, 2011).

15. Carol J. Adams, "The Book," https://caroljadams.com/spom-the-book. http://caroljadams.com/spom-the-book/.

16. Ibid.

17. "Position of the American Dietetic Association: Vegetarian Diets," *J. Am. Diet. Assoc.* 109, no. 7 (July 2009): 1266–1282.

18. See in particular these three studies: M. Thorogood, J. Mann, P. Appleby, and K. McPherson, "Risk of Death from Cancer and Ischaemic Heart Disease in Meat and Non-Meat

Eaters," *Br. Med. J.* 308 (1994): 1667–1670; J. Chang-Claude, R. Frentzel-Beyme, and U. Eilber, "Mortality Patterns of German Vegetarians after 11 Years of Follow-Up," *Epidemiology* 3 (1992): 395–401; and J. Chang-Claude and R. Frentzel-Beyme, "Dietary and Lifestyle Determinants of Mortality among German Vegetarians," *Int. J. Epidemiol.* 22 (1993): 228–236.

19. Joanne L. Slavin and Beate Lloyd, "Health Benefits of Fruits and Vegetables," *Adv. Nutr.* 3, no. 4 (July 6, 2012): 506–516, doi:10.3945/an.112.002154.

20. R. L. Phillips, "Role of Lifestyle and Dietary Habits in Risk of Cancer among Seventh-Day Adventists," *Cancer Res.* 35 (1975): 3513–3522.

21. W. C. Roberts, "Twenty Questions on Atherosclerosis," *Proceedings* (Baylor University Medical Center) 13, no. 2 (2000): 139–143.

Chapter Eight

Awareness

What We Do to Animals

AWARENESS

I have argued essentially that ethical veganism is an expression of virtue. In my view, using animals for food is a disgraceful practice. The practice of using animals for food is intrinsically wrong. Midgley argues that "some consequences are not just a matter of chance. Acts that are bad in themselves can be expected to have bad effects of a particular kind that is not just accidental."[1] As she points out, for example, lying destroys trust in human relationships; similarly, using sheep brains as cattle feed, not surprisingly, caused the infamously named "mad cow disease." I hope to have shown that using animals for food is another great example of this notion. Earlier, I discussed how, based on many studies, health science consistently shows that eating animal products is bad for human health, while plant-based diets are healthful and help lower the risk of many diseases. In what follows, I want to take the time to take a closer look at the act itself; namely, I want to describe what is involved in eating animals, showing that it is an intrinsically bad practice.

It is true that nowadays we need not go too far to see what happens in the world. YouTube and other online platforms make it easy to see, for example, the way animals are treated by the meat industry. There are many videos on the internet, especially videos filmed undercover, showing the inside of industrial farms and slaughterhouses, where farmed animals often endure shocking abuse. And there is a large literature, as well as videos, about the process of turning animals into food. One of the most heartbreaking videos is that of male baby chicks being ground alive.[2] Timothy Pachirat's *Every*

Twelve Seconds is one of the most neutral and detailed accounts of the operations of "reputable" slaughterhouses.[3] Pachirat describes stomach-twisting facts about standard practices of the industry. Such descriptions are very important for the acquisition of virtue; unfortunately these very descriptions are ignored or intentionally obscured. Most people who live in affluent societies, where eating animals is a predominant practice, have lost touch with nature. A virtue-based approach to animal ethics suggests that we should not ignore these facts. We should also have direct experience with animals to understand their moral worth. This will enable us to empathize with animals and develop compassion. The purpose of describing the process required to go from animal to meat, I believe, speaks for itself and should highlight why using animals for food is disgraceful and in nearly all cases callous.

There are many factors we must consider. First, livestock and pet breeders use artificial insemination and forced breeding to give birth to millions of animals. Dairymen separate cows from their children so their milk can be collected and sold, while the calves are slaughtered for veal. Veal calves—as the industry terms baby cows—are killed early in life when their flesh is still pale. They are given an anemic diet and kept in the dark so their flesh never turns red. Most animals are born and raised in cages, or in ranges where they are shipped to processing plants where they are killed. But meat does not grow on trees. To obtain meat, animal bodies are cut into pieces, packaged, and shipped to supermarkets where they are sold, euphemistically labeled as beef, pork, drumsticks, and so on, so as to hide as much as possible the fact that they are the mutilated body parts of animals. Far from being an appeal to emotion, this reveals how squalid it is to raise animals with the intention of killing them and using their flesh, skin, fluids, and the rest. Animals are creatures that are capable of flourishing, but their lives are destroyed by human craving for meat; this inflicts pain on them, prevents their flourishing and human flourishing as well. Animals used for food are docile animals that are killed. Their body parts are sold as food.

Some people know or are aware of all these facts about the meat industry but do not conclude that veganism is obligatory. While I find this disheartening, I want to point out that this is the very reason why it is important to acquire the virtues. It seems hard to say that a compassionate, just, temperate, and magnanimous person would participate in a practice that destroys the lives of animals on the grounds of taste or perhaps tradition. Not surprisingly, however, the current state of things is due to the influence of consequentialist and deontological ethics, which, as I pointed out, de-emphasizes feeling, relationship, and what Midgley calls the "yuck factor." Whether at the industrial level or in a small setting, the lives of animals are precious, and therefore exploiting them or destroying them for the enjoyment of food or other purposes is contrary to the virtues.

Thus, my argument is that VE, alongside care and feminist ethics, can make a cumulative case for ethical veganism. VE suggests that humans have the function of acting in accordance with reason, and this activity leads to flourishing—that is, it leads to a good life for human beings. A good life is characterized by noble actions guided by virtues such as compassion, empathy, justice, temperance, magnanimity, and more. These virtues open our eyes and our hearts to a reality that other moral theories are incapable of doing. They demonstrate facts about our relationship and our treatment of animals that we might miss if we look at the world only in terms of what is beneficial to the greatest number or which rights belong to which individuals. Indeed, using animals for food and other purposes is typically squalid. Even in those cases where animals are "treated well," the truth is that those animals will lose their lives, will be separated from their children, and will be turned into food or products that are not essential to us. Most of these processes involve physical or mental suffering, boredom, isolation, and depression. With regard to food, it is inevitable that the process involves blood and death.

The animals that meat eaters consume are highly sensitive and intelligent creatures. It is no longer a matter of debate that creatures like pigs and chickens have elaborate social systems. They are peaceful and playful, and I don't believe it is anthropomorphism to say that they enjoy their existence. We know this because those animals are incapable of expressing the same passion for life when confined in pens or crowded spaces and forced to live away from their natural environment, offspring, and friends. At this point, there are hundreds of testimonies of people who experienced firsthand the horror of slaughterhouses and factory farms. They all tell the same tale of animals suffering and, most importantly, their own negative experiences of witnessing the fear in the eyes of animals that are about to be killed. It is not a mystery that humans share the same concerns about life and death. We value our freedom, our ability to have a social life, and we have a strong desire to live free from suffering. It is not inconsistent or implausible, then, that we should value these aspects in the lives of animals. VE argues that a life devoid of unnecessary blood dripping from the corpses of animals, devoid of millions of animals artificially brought into existence, is a life that is beneficial to us, and thus a virtuous life. Ethical veganism, therefore, is the natural expression of virtue.

What I outlined above marks a salient distinction between various moral theories. Namely, VE, unlike other theories, argues that we need to acquire moral virtues that function as lenses through which we clearly see that animals are creatures that value their own existence and with whom we share relevant moral characteristics. This is a hard point to argue, but I tried to explain that possessing the virtues makes one see what is wrong with using animals for food, clothing, and entertainment; exploiting animals involves activities that are contrary to compassion, justice, temperance, and greatness of soul, and in so doing we undermine our moral integrity. Again, the point of VE is not to give people a series of rules or prescriptions that must be followed, though this is not to say that a virtuous individual could not offer general prescriptions that conform to the actions and sentiments of a noble character. However, VE, as I understand it as a commonsense theory, suggests that without the virtues we are morally lost and in the hands of impersonal rules that will not lead to a happy life. Furthermore, VE suggests that morality involves more than just calculation. It involves learning about others, in this case about the life of animals. Learning what animals are like enables us to see that they are creatures whose existence matters. This is not true for everyone. But as I argue, this is due to a distorted view of morality that emphasizes rights and duties instead of feeling and relationship. When we take the time to realize that a cow is not an object that we may use for our benefit, but rather a creature capable of being happy, who exists for her own sake, by the very definition of the virtues we cannot possibly regard her as a walking hunk of meat waiting to be killed, milked, eaten, and used for clothing. The idea is not that we refrain from killing her, but that a fair, compassionate, and empathetic individual by definition sees a cow (or any other animal) as a precious being endowed with feelings and many important capacities that we recognize as morally important. A virtuous individual, therefore, does not regard animals as food any more or any less than he regards a human baby as food.

SHOULD WE ALL BECOME VEGANS?

But perhaps there is a more difficult question: "Why vegan and not vegetarian?" Why does VE, when properly understood, lead to veganism? For example, why is it wrong to take the milk of a cow and drink it or use it to make cheese or take the eggs of a chicken for food? Suppose these animals are not slaughtered and live "happy" lives. In the first place, such is not the scenario that is in question here. Cows and chickens are domesticated animals that humans long ago decided to dominate and possess for food, clothing, and more. A virtuous individual takes these facts into consideration and realizes that cows and chickens are truly happy if they are not exploited. The fact that many people do not see the wrongness of a so-called happy cow "donating" her milk is because many people have been disciplined into thinking that human beings have the right to exploit animals. Naturally, if we start with such a presupposition, we will find no fault in the idea of taking milk from a cow or eggs from a chicken. Conversely, a virtuous individual realizes that a cow is not something that we have the right to possess and that a cow's milk is not human food but a baby cow's food. Cow's milk is in reality a bodily secretion not meant for human consumption.

Returning to the idea of compassion, I argued that a compassionate individual is concerned about the well-being of all living things. He respects all creatures because all have a dignity and deserve moral respect. So, one may object that since plants are also exploited and used as food, it would seem to follow that a virtuous individual would also avoid eating them. In other words, why is eating plants compassionate but eating animal by-products is not? I think the answer starts by considering that the actions of a virtuous individual are measured according to the given circumstances. Compassion is applied in different degrees according to the particular living organism. This means that while a compassionate individual has moral respect for all living things, the degree of respect is different for different beings and different situations.

Considering the cognitive capacities that animals have, and considering the horrendous practices required to turn animals into food, it is reasonable to say that a compassionate individual avoids using animals because it causes pain and suffering to them. In this case, a compassionate individual may consistently eat plants but avoid eating animals and their by-products because using plants does not require those painful practices that I outlined above. So, it might turn out that plants have certain important cognitive capacities, that they are sentient; but it is reasonable to say that it is more compassionate to use them than to exploit animals who exhibit a higher degree of sentience and conscious experience of the world. Namely, unlike plants, animals are social creatures possessing cognitive capacities, by virtue of which they experience the world. We see that they are not mere objects but beings that experience feelings of fear and joy, and that have relationships with friends and with their own offspring.

THE LINK BETWEEN VIRTUE AND VEGANISM

What link is there between VE and ethical veganism? I suppose we may frame this question by considering two further points: (1) Given the virtues, what should we do? In what way are the virtues capable of guiding us to veganism? (2) Is it all about avoiding cruelty? If we treat animals with respect—"humanely," as they say—are we morally permitted to, say, own animals or drink the occasional freshly squeezed milk or eat eggs or wear wool?

1. The action guiding is one of those aspects in ethics that strikes me as being portrayed as the most difficult and that is a deal breaker for VE. Expanding on Hursthouse's discussion about this,[4] I have to mention that deontology and consequentialism, which are typically regarded as great action guiding theories, stand in the same need of an explanation for moral action guiding as VE. At any rate, the criticism that VE fails to give moral

guidance stems from an approach to VE with the same standards used for non-VE theories. That is, it is a type of category mistake to ask about action guiding of VE, like asking whether a chair is compassionate. Yet it is not entirely out of the question for VE to direct us in right moral directions.

Because VE is focused on the good and excellence of the individual, its action guiding power is possessed by it in a different form, internally. Formulaic theories are those that offer a procedure, such as the utilitarian calculus or the universalizability principle leading to categorical imperatives, to determine the right action; such theories are purported to yield decisions that are right actions and at the same time moral actions. VE has no formula per se, so the action guiding force is internal to the agent rather than external. The acquisition of the virtues creates an individual who by nature makes good and right decisions and arguably rational decisions. In the literature, this is a serious point of contention against VE, but not a correct one. To work this out with an analogy, think about a well-educated individual having a discussion. He listens to his interlocutors, allows them to express their position, and then politely responds. An ill-educated individual, on the other hand, may not be so polite to allow others to talk or may not use the principle of charity in a discussion. Now, the idea is that a well-educated individual is one who enjoys having polite discussions because he possesses certain virtues that make him a polite and respectful individual.

So, properly understood, VE suggests that a virtuous individual possesses a good character that leads her in the right moral direction. The issue about whether VE can be a viable action guiding theory is exacerbated by lifeboat hypotheticals. For instance, a critic may ask, "Granted, compassion and fairness are noble aspects of one's character, but how do you deal with this and that situation?" As mentioned before, we must realize that every theory is open to this criticism, but this is not simply a *tu quoque* fallacy. Consider deontology, which I find plausible. For instance, I help you because I have a sense of duty and not because I have an ulterior motive—or, I do the right thing for the right reasons. So, for example, I never lie, because not lying is a duty that requires that I act from a good will. But then what should I do if you were hiding in my house from a hypothetical killer and the killer asked me if I had seen you? Should I tell the truth according to the imperative "never lie" and risk your life, or should I lie to protect you? In such a case, a deontologist is morally paralyzed. But VE is an entirely different approach because, arguably, a virtuous individual is caring and compassionate and would lie every time in such hypothetical circumstances to save another's life. But what's important here is to understand that there is not a formula that says, in such-and-such circumstance, tell the truth or lie or what have you. Right action is not one that occurs independently of an individual's state of mind—one that shows respect for life, concern about justice, benevolence, empathy, and friendship—which moves the agent to perform a proper action that is appropriate in given circumstances. In the specific instance the circumstances are that we can thrive on an exclusively vegan diet and so do not need to exploit animals.

A virtuous individual is not preoccupied about which action is right and which method or formula will lead to the right action. This is the sense in which VE is action guiding: An honest individual is one that never lies unless lying is for a good cause. For example, such an individual, having the virtue of honesty but also of compassion, might find it appropriate to avoid telling a child that her mother was raped and brutally murdered. The point is that a virtuous individual, unlike a deontologist or a consequentialist, need not worry about calculating the right action because what is right is dictated, so to speak, by the virtues.

Now the question of how to move from the virtues to veganism requires a few steps. But how does this work? When I think about people, I do not think of them as potential food. VE suggests that I consider my feelings and assess the specific situation when I interact with others. Once again, in terms of universalizability, my feelings toward others are objective because I objectively recognize a moral worth in others. So while my decisions may change according to particular circumstances, the fact that others have moral value is a fact about nature that is unchanging. A virtuous individual recognizes that others are valuable individuals deserving attention and moral respect. As we recognize our value, we recognize the value of others. I believe that this cannot be put any more saliently than it was by Albert Schweitzer:

> Just as in my own will-to-live there is a yearning for my life, and for that mysterious exultation of the will-to-live which is called pleasure, and terror in face of annihilation and that injury to the will-to-live which is called pain; so the same obtains in all the will-to-live around me, equally whether it can express itself to my comprehension or whether it remains unvoiced.[5]

It is not the case that I respect others because they are rational beings or because I want to promote the highest aggregative good. Rather, I respect them because I recognize their uniqueness and that their existence is valuable to them as my existence is to me. A compassionate and fair character, in other words, enables me to have reverence for life itself and recognize that animals are not objects that can be exploited, but rather are highly sensitive creatures that have a yearning for their lives.

2. Consequently, I do not see animals as things that I might eat or use. So ethical veganism is not only a matter of avoiding cruelty. I see animals as they are: They are individuals, siblings, mothers, fathers, and friends; they are beings that care for one another, that enjoy each other's company. These considerations do not stem from a principle of right or what might lead to the promotion of the greatest good for the greatest number. Rather, I acknowl-

edge what animals are as living beings by observing them and learning about them and listening to them. They do not behave like food, smell like food, or look like food. They are cute, playful, funny, aggressive, affectionate, dangerous, and much more.

Learning about animals makes us realize that they have interesting social lives. Like humans, animals enjoy the company of their siblings, friends, and parents; many animals also enjoy human company. Animals have to be turned into food. This involves no pretty sights or smells. In this process, there are forcible appropriation of animals, forcible reproduction, lacerations of the skin, castration, debeaking, blood and other fluids flowing out of their bodies, broken bones, an experience of fear and pain, and unpleasant odors, just to mention a few crude events involved in the transformation of animals into food. The horrendous sights, sounds, and odors caused by the death of an animal are, I argue, atrocious events. Consider that such animals, very plausibly, do not desire to be turned into food. Also interesting to note is that unless we purchase their body parts in a supermarket, conveniently cut into welcoming shapes and packaged, most people would feel distress were they themselves required to kill and turn animals into food. Furthermore, an equally important consideration, though not an essential one for the case, is that the human body requires no consumption of animal flesh or animal derivatives. So, because animals are individuals with intrinsic moral worth that exist for their own sake, I also realize that it is unjust, cruel, and uncaring to use them in any kind of way. Furthermore, considering that animals such as cows and chickens have been domesticated for the very purpose of being eaten and used in various practices of human existence, consuming milk, using wool, and other practices that some might label as "humane" are in disaccord with the virtues.

To spell this out, as in the case of our relationship with other humans, a compassionate, just, temperate, and empathetic individual does not regard animals as food or clothing or entertainment. VE does not suggest that we avoid exploiting and eating humans or animals only because we should avoid cruelty; also, we do not refrain from eating or using people or animals because we are interested in maximizing utility or because we must follow certain fixed rules dictated by reason. Rather, we respect others because we recognize their intrinsic moral worth, which is evinced by our capacity to relate to them and have relationships. Consequently, I recognize that even drinking a mother's milk is unvirtuous, unless she is my mother and I am at an age that requires that I drink breast milk. The point is that avoiding cruelty is not enough to realize which practices are immoral. Only through the virtues, especially compassion, temperance, fairness, and magnanimity, can we realize that most of the practices and attitudes toward animals that we consider humane are in fact morally bankrupt.

Therefore, having learned important facts about us and about the lives of animals, VE's approach cannot be vague or yield equally possible courses of action. If VE wants me to be a fair individual, for example, once I realize that animals do not belong to us, yet are forcibly impregnated, held captive, and arbitrarily used, I know that what is involved in the process of turning animals into food is in no sense just. Similarly, VE suggests that we be empathetic and compassionate. Empathy is a virtue that enables us to fully understand the situation of another being. Compassion is the sympathetic and genuine concern for the feelings of others, especially for their suffering and misfortune. Now, having realized that animals exist for their own benefit and that it is not their purpose or wish to be imprisoned and turned into food, a practice that inflicts pain and suffering, we then realize that using animals does not conform to virtue, and therefore regarding animals as things that we can eat is uncompassionate and unfair. Notice that an evaluation of these important virtues enables us to address the second point—that is, whether it is morally permissible within a VE framework to *use* animals if we avoid making them suffer. The emphasis on the word *use* is important here. For, considering the virtues, using others for our benefit the way we use animals for food, clothing, research, and entertainment is a sign of lack of virtue. In most cases, we might believe it morally permissible to use animals if we regard animals as objects of utility or objects possessing rights. VE suggests that we consider whether our actions that involve turning animals into food, clothing, and subjects of scientific research and entertainment are noble actions. As I hope to have shown, such actions are due to intemperance, and disregard for the function of animals as beings whose lives matter to them. Consequently, the point of view of certain ways of using animals are humane.

REACHING PEOPLE IN NON-MANIPULATIVE WAYS

In order to shake off the idea that animals are our property and food, it is necessary to see where such a false idea originates. In my view, it is an idea produced by the systematically manipulative instruction of society, especially by those institutions that have an economic interest in the meat and dairy, entertainment, and fashion industries. Thus, I want to discuss what forms of non-manipulative instruction may succeed in reaching people and perhaps what steps are necessary to avert this manipulative process. First, I want to point out the specifics of manipulating people. There are, I believe, mechanisms that subvert our opposition to animal exploitation. The aspect of VE that I emphasize is knowledge of what is relevant in a particular aspect of moral life. I argue that it is precisely understanding these mechanisms that enables us to acquire the virtues. VE suggests that we must acquire certain moral character traits that will enable us to live well, and as a result will enable us to regard animals as beings existing for their own sake. This in its turn can show us that ethical veganism is an expression of virtuous character. When we approach animal ethics from virtue, we realize that using animals for our benefit is an expression of vice or lack of virtue. The dominance of deontological and consequentialist ethics has shaped our understanding of our relationship with animals. As I pointed out, such moral approaches have discounted the importance of empathy, compassion, temperance, and, overall, the importance of what it is to be a great-souled individual. Thus a question is prompted: What prevents us from having sympathy and compassion toward animals so that we oppose animal exploitation and embrace ethical veganism? My answer is that the meat-and-dairy industry, alongside hunting, scientific research, and entertainment businesses have established very powerful mechanisms to subvert and override our moral feelings of sympathy toward animals.

Tom Regan questions whether in morality our emotions alone can move us in the direction of opposing animal exploitation. In this particular passage, he questions whether care ethics can "go far enough."[6] He writes,

> What are the resources within the ethic of care that can move people to consider the ethics of their dealings within individuals who *stand outside* the existing circle of their valued interpersonal relationships? . . . Unless we supplement the ethic of care with some other motivating source—some other grounding of our moral judgment—we run the grave risk that our ethic will be excessively conservative and will blind us to those obligations we have to people for whom we are indifferent.
>
> Nowhere, perhaps, is this possibility more evident than in the case of our moral dealings with non-human animals. The plain fact is, most people do not care very much about what happens to them. . . .
>
> And thus it is that a feminist ethic that is *limited to an ethic of care* will, I think, be unable to illuminate the moral significance of the idea that we (human) animals are not superior to all the animals.[7]

And Peter Singer argues that the best way to make us realize that we should accept equal consideration for animals and thus oppose animal exploitation is the utilitarian idea of preference. Like Regan, Singer believes that reason, not emotion, is necessary for us to see the wrongness of animal exploitation. In fact, he writes that

> altruistic impulses once limited to one's kin and one's own group might be extended to a wider circle by reasoning creatures who can see that they and their kin are one group among others, and from an impartial point of view no more important than others.[8]

Singer and Regan here argue that people lack sympathy for animals. What I find interesting is that neither denies the value of sympathy. Regan says it is "a plain fact" that people do not care about animals, and for Singer it is a *natural fact*. In my view, people do not care about animals because they are taught to do so by manipulative mechanisms created by society to undermine sympathy toward animals who stand outside our circle of care. What seems to be infelicitous about our relationship with animals is that we have to be taught to exploit them, to use them as food, or in general that they exist for our own benefit. Early in our lives, we have to be slowly habituated to regard animals as food. Animals are typically fed to children in forms that do not remotely resemble animals, such as mush or cute shapes, such as nuggets or things labeled as "happy meals." It is not surprising that people are naturally repulsed by the view of blood and death. Children in particular are kept uninformed of the process required to turn animals into their "happy meals." Moreover, children's books make sure to distort children's reality by presenting animals as happy friends of, say, Farmer Joe's, rather than showing them amassed in cages inside factory farms. Not surprisingly, children are not taught that burgers and steaks are former body parts of the same cute cow they see in their book where the cows appear so peaceful and content. There is a clear mechanism that disconnects children's understanding of the lives of animals and prevents the acquisition of important moral virtues such as compassion and fairness. It is interesting to read a few comments about this topic in a public forum. The following comments are anecdotal but nonetheless seem to corroborate the point of common sense as well as scientific studies showing that when certain virtues are acquired, animals appear to us for what they are and cease to be regarded as food. Most people are aware, more or less, that meat comes from animals, but the actual process is not easily grasped and taken to heart. In most cases, such discussions are avoided or downplayed by caregivers:

> Mandi Roberts: I always had an awareness that meat came from animals, but I wasn't aware of the actual process. I'm from a family of big meat eaters so eating meat, or my dad's gratuitous gory rendition of killing animals, was always looked upon with a twisted type of humor. It wasn't until I was around 7, that I realized what animals actually went through and that I didn't have to eat meat to survive (though my dad would often react as though your opinion was idiotic—or frankly you were, for not eating meat). I remember talking about it as a child, but it was quickly swept under the carpet as we were repeatedly told "you'll get what you're given," "we weren't as lucky as you in my day," and "you'll eat it or wear it." Discussions weren't to be had growing up!

Rebecca Coplon: My son was about 3 when he got the idea that chicken was, well, made of chicken, but about 4 when he put two and two together and realized he was EATING A CHICKEN! He has never loved eating meat since that realization, and takes short forays into the idea of being a vegetarian. He's nearly 12 now. Even in Minecraft, he tends to be a vegetarian, and resists killing the little digital beasts to get meat or leather.

Anita Holton: I'm sure my kids realized around age 4 or so, but I don't think they really grasped what this meant. They understood that chicken nuggets were made from chickens and hamburgers were made from cows. I think it was only as they got older that they could empathize that animals want to live and enjoy their lives and families like humans. At age 8 my middle son decided to become a vegetarian. I supported him and my oldest son and I joined him. Eventually my husband and youngest son decided to become vegetarians too. After 4 years of a vegetarian diet we transitioned to a vegan diet. Note, this was my son that started us on this journey. No-one was forced to be a vegetarian or eventually become vegan. My kids are now 12, 16, and 19. They have remained committed to their choice.

Greg C Neumayer: When and should we help our kids understand that eating meat involves killing animals? I think we all should be aware of where our meat comes from—this means having a good idea what a beef or chicken farm looks like from the field to the bag. If I'm not comfortable with the process, I shouldn't eat it. If I want to turn a blind eye or remain in ignorance, what's happening in my head? I'm wanting to enjoy something without knowledge of its true cost or impact. Pure selfishness, if I indulge it.

Erica Challis: At around 3, for our son. He stopped eating meat because it was made of animals, he said. At six, he still hasn't eaten meat since he was three.

Subha Thankaraj: I was showing my 3 and half year old daughter the video of dairy product factory. The video was halfway, around where the packaging of milk in bottles was shown, when she asked, "So, now do they give this milk to baby cow?" I replied, "No. It's transported to supermarkets and we buy it." Then, she asked "So, what do baby cows drink?"

Germaine Cecil: When I was 7 I was actively seeking answers about the animals and how I managed to eat them without harming them, once I realized that they had to be killed for me to eat . . . and the conditions of being force fed and so forth I stopped eating meat. . . . I've been vegetarian ever since.[9]

What I want to point out about experience is that at a tender age, people eat what their caregivers feed them. Many children, however, realize that there is something funny about eating meat. In many cases, that curiosity is not given the right attention or the facts are hidden from children. Most children show empathy and are deeply moved by their compassion and realize that there is something fundamentally wrong with eating animals. In fact, it is my view that this stage of life is critical for acquiring the virtues. Unfortunately, later in life other factors get in the way. Younger people show a natural concern for others and consequently reject the idea of eating animals; they "significantly agreed more with the moral reason and with the environmental reason. People ages 41–60 significantly agreed more with the health reason. There are significant differences across generations as to why people choose to live a vegetarian lifestyle."[10]

A recent study concluded that vegetarianism in children ages six to ten is based on moral understanding of motivations, such as animal welfare, rather than personal motivations. The vegetarian children included in this study gave moral reasons that evince virtuous feelings. Conversely, children who ate meat did not acknowledge such feelings at all.[11] What prevents non-vegetarian children from empathizing with animals?

The work of Dr. Melanie Joy helps to understand the false instruction I am referring to here, and it answers the question above. According to Joy, people are conditioned to eat certain animals. In most cases, people do not even know that they have a choice. She calls this belief system "carnism," which in her words is

> the invisible belief system, or ideology, that conditions us to eat certain animals. It is the opposite of veganism. We tend to label only those ideologies that fall outside the norm, as though the dominant culture doesn't have a belief system. For instance, we tend to assume that only vegans and vegetarians bring their beliefs to the dinner table, but that's not the case. When eating animals is not a necessity for survival—which is the case in much of the world today—then it is a choice. And choices always stem from beliefs.[12]

As mentioned earlier, when children experience food and express concern about eating meat, sometimes by using the "yuck factor" or by fully articulating their compassionate views, they are frequently denied the choice of being vegetarians by their caregivers or they are assured by their caregivers that there is nothing wrong with eating animals. It seems to me that when children's feelings of disgust or compassion emerge, and they are allowed to explore such feelings, the children act on a deep and compassionate instinct and avoid eating animals or using anything that was obtained from animals.

The study I cite above also showed that the main barrier to vegetarianism among children is their caregivers' influence on their children. Children are conditioned to follow the eating habits and choices of adults. Typically, if caregivers eat animals, their children are often unaware, or they are intentionally kept unaware, that eating a plant-based diet is a possibility.

Another mechanism that in some cases prevents people from living according to their deepest feelings of compassion toward animals is, arguably, religion. I want to make it clear from the start that I am not arguing that religion is deliberately deceiving or suggesting that belief in a god is illusory or that religion is inherently counterproductive for morality. Rather, I want to point out that religions, insofar as social phenomena, regardless of whether a god or gods exist, are affected by social trends just like everything else in society. So it is not surprising that the prevalent religious view accommodates exploitation of animals. The Bible, for example, would seem to speak in favor of ethical veganism, as Genesis 1:29–30 states the following:

> Then God said, "I give you every seed-bearing plant on the face of the whole earth and every tree that has fruit with seed in it. They will be yours for food. And to all the beasts of the earth and all the birds in the sky and all the creatures that move along the ground—everything that has the breath of life in it—I give every green plant for food." And it was so. [13]

This passage clearly states that animals were not created as "human food"—and I agree with this—but rather as creatures that exist for their own sake, who have a dignity and are morally very different from plants. Animals eat plants, fruits, and seeds, just like humans. And in Genesis 1:1–2:3 animals are created before humans and are regarded as good independent of their relations to human beings. But these passages are seldom cited or known by Christians, who actually know of passages where animals are offered to humans by God as food. Interestingly, the Qur'an also describes animals as morally important beings that, like humans, and unlike plants, form communities. The book describes them in a very dignified way, to the extent that animals will in the end know God. Animals here are far from being viewed as human food or property:

> There is not an animal that lives on the earth, nor a being that flies on its wings, but they form communities like you. Nothing have we omitted from the Book, and they all shall be gathered to their Lord in the end. [14]

But once again, it is understandable that most Muslims prefer other passages of the Qur'an where meat is food. But my point about religion, again, is not a general critique. In fact, I believe that properly understood, most religions have the resources to defend ethical veganism. My point is that there are many interpretations of the same concept within the same religion and there are also religions, such as Jainism, that teach reverence for life and veganism. Jains, for example, are typically vegetarians. And the Seventh-Day Adventist Church, a Protestant Christian denomination, has a reading of the Bible according to which eating meat is not encouraged: "We believe God calls us to care for our bodies, treating them with the respect a divine creation deserves. Gluttony and excess, even of something good, can be detrimental to our health."[15] Incidentally, the view of the Seventh-Day Adventist Church encapsulates my earlier argument that eating animal products marks a sign of intemperance, though my view does not appeal to a divinity.

Language is possibly the most powerful manipulative mechanism. It is obvious by watching commercials or reading meat trade or hunting journals, or just by visiting the meat section of any supermarket, that terminology used to describe animals and animal products is suspiciously euphemistic. I say suspiciously because I argue that language about animals is specifically designed to divorce certain images from animals—images such as slaughter, blood, imprisonment, torture, exploitation, suffering, and more. I shall mention a few examples. A typical expression in relation to meat dishes is about the "juices" or how "juicy" a piece of meat is; however, meat does not contain juice. The liquid dripping from a piece of meat is blood. Butcher shops nowadays are almost all known as "meat markets." Slaughterhouses prefer to be called "meat plants" or even "meat factories" to hide the fact that animals there are, well, slaughtered. Not to mention that the meat industry uses terms such as "beef," "pork," "white meat," "flank steak," "round," "mountain oysters," and many other euphemisms to refer to cow flesh, pig flesh, the breast of a chicken, the rear end of a cow, animal testicles, and so on. Similarly, vivisectionists prefer to use terms such as "dispatch," or "terminate," or "sacrifice" instead of "kill." Hunting is usually regarded as a sport, although the activity itself is likened to agriculture; hunters favor terms such as "harvesting" to refer to killing animals by shooting them.

And to top it all off, this type of deliberately deceitful language pervades society through and through with the aid and persuasive power of the media. It appears that TV shows and movies try to give a negative connotation to vegetables, vegetarians, and vegans, while they praise what Dr. Joy refers to as "carnism" as well as animal-based diets. Perhaps one of the male-dominant mechanisms of oppression perpetrated by language that Carol Adams denounces is exemplified by the way women, men, and food are portrayed by the media: Meat is strong and salad is weak. Women continue to be viewed as weak individuals who eat weak food; women in the media are typically "salad eaters" while men are strong "meat eaters." As an example, in the popular sitcom *Two and a Half Men*, the main character, Charlie, played by Charlie Sheen, is the stereotypical male—a gambler, drinker, womanizer, who enjoys eating meat and smoking cigars. In one episode, Charlie is dating a woman, also portrayed as the stereotypical female—a submissive, long-haired ballerina—who has the preposterous idea of trying to change Charlie into a "better" man by taking him to a vegan restaurant. The result is disastrous, as Charlie defies his date by shouting that he cannot stand having to eat "medallions of bean curd in lawnmower sauce"[16] like a woman.

The point is always the same: Meat eating is praised with a good/positive connotation, it is generally associated with ideas of strength and masculinity, and it is synonymous with reason and righteousness; meanwhile veganism or even vegetarianism is undermined and ridiculed as associated with femininity, and femininity is portrayed as synonymous with irrationality, emotiveness, daintiness, and overall silliness. Films, magazine articles, TV shows, comedies, talk shows, and more depict vegans negatively. They are always soft-character, bunny-like, salad eaters or obnoxious individuals who bother other people, feel superior, or want to save the world. The very term "vegan" is nowadays synonymous with a restrictive or cult-like diet, so that it is viewed as just another diet among hundreds, and the actual moral question of our treatment of animals becomes obscured. My point here is that animal exploitation thrives not because humans do not have a natural bond with animals, but in spite of it. People are deliberately manipulated by a system of exploitation, which comprises scientific research, meat and dairy industries, hunting, and the food industry. If we are constantly given these messages, we cannot be properly informed about the lives of animals, and therefore cannot sympathize with them.

What forms of instruction, then, can inform in a non-manipulative way and help people overcome the false idea that animals are human property and food? It is a rather complicated issue that has to come to terms with multimillion-dollar industries that hold sway over government and the media. But the first step is to realize the subversive ways used by the media to discipline people out of their empathy toward animals. One answer is to become more involved in moral education and move in the direction of VE instead of the prevalent view of morality that teaches us about rights, utility, or about detached principles and rules. Informing the public might also involve a new direction for academic philosophers toward a more practical way of teaching and doing philosophy. After all, I believe that the moral mistake of exploiting animals stems from a lack of virtue and an abundance of vices. For example, besides indifference to the suffering of animals, intemperance is manifested in people's obsession with food, regardless of whether or not such food comes through the suffering of animals. Self-indulgence is also manifested in the insistence on consuming animal products of all kinds, whether they are consumed as food or clothing. Viable methods of instruction will require a demand of clear information from government and the media. This may start, in my view, by educating children about the lives of animals and the procedures involved in turning animals into food, shoes, and wallets, as well as the use of animals in scientific research. But most importantly it will show examples, through literature, the arts, and entertainment, of the lives of vegans as they really are—morally consistent and dietarily fulfilled—and the lives of animals as they are—that is, beings that have important moral characteristics, beings that want to exist for their own sake and not for the sake of humans.

The issue of tobacco is similar, in my view, in that it is an immoral business that thrives on misinformation and the intemperance of millions of people who indulge in smoking cigarettes. In 2009, the Family Smoking Prevention and Tobacco Control Act was signed into law and required, among many other provisions, the display of color graphics and texts that depict the negative consequences of smoking. I am not suggesting that we should require photos on packages of meat of animals being slaughtered (though it is not an entirely bad idea). However, despite the message and the images and our knowledge of the lethal consequences of cigarette smoking, people continue to smoke, although far fewer of them than in the past. This is once again due to the lack of virtue and the continuing promotion of smoking by the tobacco industry through movies and celebrity usage. In a similar fashion, both the meat and dairy industry and the tobacco industry work very hard to make immoral practices, such as the exploitation of animals and the sale of a lethal drug, seem necessary in our lives.

I want to make a final point about language, morality, and information. Earlier I mentioned a YouTube video of a food demonstrator in a supermarket offering samples of sausage to passing customers. When the customers sought to purchase the product, the demonstrator would remove a piglet from a box and pretend to drop the cute squirming piglet into what seemed like a meat grinder. The reaction of all the customers was the same: They were shocked and appalled at the cruelty and cold heart of the demonstrator who pretended to throw the piglet into the meat grinder without hesitation. This predicament occurs while most of the customers are still chewing their sausage. But then, why are the customers shocked? By what are they appalled? Also, why are many meat eaters and leather wearers opposed to animal exploitation? Usually people say that they are against inhumane treatment of animals. But what makes them say that a certain treatment is inhumane? Why do some people bother at all worrying about whether or not the treatment that animals receive is humane? If one has such worries, why eat animals or wear their skin in the first place? Such conflicting attitudes, I believe, evince a schizophrenic moral attitude and a truncated expression of our moral feelings of compassion, fairness, and benevolence for non-human animals.[17] The point of moral education should be to nurture these feelings and enable us to apply them consistently in harmony with reason. As I have pointed out, one is truly and fully compassionate when feelings of compassion are consistently directed toward all animals, not just those close to us. Also, a fair individual is one who, having acquired a just, moral character, is fair in all circumstances. The compassionate and fair-minded individual is a great-souled individual who feels sympathy for all animals and avoids exploiting them because it is unfair to do so. In other words, a virtuous individual understands that animals are not our food, and therefore chooses to be an ethical vegan.

NOTES

1. Midgley, "Biotechnology and Monstrosity," 8.
2. A search on YouTube leads to numerous videos of baby male chicks ground alive. The one I watched is "Egg Industry Grinds Millions of Baby Chicks Alive," https://www.youtube.com/watch?v=BQ5qAfyUuWE by HoTvid HD. For a number of reasons, these videos are often removed. This particular video was still up as of June 2018. In the event it is removed, there are many others showing similar content.
3. See Pachirat, *Every Twelve Seconds: Industrialized Slaughter and the Politics of Sight* (New Haven, CT: Yale University Press, 2013).
4. Here I refer to Rosalind Hursthouse, "Normative Virtue Ethics," in *How Should One Live?* ed. Roger Crisp (Oxford: Oxford University Press, 1996), 19–33.
5. Schweitzer, "The Ethic of Reverence for Life," 32–33.
6. Regan, *The Thee Generation: Reflections of the Coming Revolution* (Philadelphia: Temple University Press, 1991), 95.
7. Ibid., 95–96.
8. Singer, *The Expanding Circle: Ethics and Sociology* (New York: Farrar, Straus, and Giroux, 1981), 134.
9. Quora.com, "When Do Kids Realize That Eating Meat Involves Killing Animals?"
10. See P. Pribis, R. C. Pencak, and T. Grajales, "Beliefs and Attitudes toward Vegetarian Lifestyle across Generations," *Nutrients* 2, no. 5 (2010): 523–531, http://doi.org/10.3390/nu2050523.
11. Karen M. Hussar and Paul L. Harris, "Children Who Choose Not to Eat Meat: A Study of Early Moral Decision-Making," *Social Development* 19, doi: 10.1111/j.1467-9507.2009.00547.
12. Joy, "Dis-ease of the Heart: The Psychology of Eating Animals," *Forks over Knives*, May 23, 2012.
13. Genesis 1:29–30.
14. Qur'an 6:38.
15. Seventh-Day Adventist Church, "Living a Healthful Life," https://www.adventist.org/en/vitality/health/.
16. "My Tongue Is Meat," *Two and a Half Men*, Episode 15, Season 3 (CBS, 2003–2015), February 27, 2006.
17. See Michael Stocker, "The Schizophrenia of Modern Ethical Theories," *Journal of Philosophy* 73 (1976).

Chapter Nine

Ethical Veganism's Beef with Cultured Meat

As human ingenuity progresses, new moral questions present themselves. In fact, technology has come to the point where human and animal parts can be grown in a laboratory, as indicated by the suggestive title—"Organs Made to Order"—of an article published in *Smithsonian Magazine*.[1] In medicine, researchers are now able to build replacement body parts from the cells of a patient. And other researchers are now able to grow burgers in a laboratory. Leaving aside the morality of growing human parts in a lab for medical use, our question is this: Is growing meat in a laboratory ethical? This question is tremendously interesting, especially to ethical vegans. Meat eaters don't seem to mind where meat comes from. The whole point is taste. If its taste is identical to "real" meat, then what's the problem with lab-grown meat? If we add that eating lab-grown meat will also save the planet, then that's like hitting the jackpot. What else do we need to know? If the question is "Is growing meat in a lab moral?" it seems that from the standpoint of meat eaters the answer is simple: Yes, it is moral! It reduces animal suffering and it saves the planet from environmental degradation. And it would seem that for the same reasons vegans would also deem the practice of lab-grown meat as moral. The aim of this book is to show that a proper understanding of the morality of the relationship between humans and non-human animals leads to ethical veganism, which means avoiding any food that comes from animals. Thus, it is interesting to see how the question of artificially grown meat squares off in this moral equation. I often heard that the day lab-grown meat becomes a reality, there would be no further qualms from vegans about eating meat. Hence, I want to explore this very idea and see how the question of producing meat in laboratories may or may not affect my argument that a good individual is one who possesses and practices certain virtues, and that ethical veganism is the embodiment of human virtues. It would seem that if no animal is disrespected or hurt, a magnanimous individual would have no objection to artificially grown meat, since no apparently cruel or unjust thing is done in producing this type of meat.

VIRTUE AND OBJECTIONS

There are obvious objections that a virtuous individual could raise. Animals have to be used, in any case, for the production of cultured meat. Namely, whether its painful or painless, animals must be reared and their cells must be taken from them in order to replicate them in a laboratory. Consequently, it would still be animal exploitation, which is what a virtuous person avoids. Also, researchers or the FDA or any other entity could argue that eating cloned meat is risk-free. They could say that lab meat is safe and not carcinogenic or capable of causing other ailments. But how could they possibly know about long-term effects? My main concern is this: If it's meat, then it's meat. That is, whether from the lab or from the farm, meat is unhealthful to humans.[2] Furthermore, it would seem that meat eaters, at least at present, do not like the idea of eating something made in a laboratory. Granted, it is possible that in the future lab-grown meat will taste exactly like the real deal and people will overcome the idea of meat that was artificially grown. At any rate, it is reasonable to believe that not all meat eaters will embrace lab-grown meat. If this is the case, by the way, the project of cloning meat is not an alternative competitor to raising animals but merely another option. It is entirely possible that it will be received as a fad and that traditional meat production will not change to the degree necessary to save the planet from the negative environmental consequences caused by raising animals.

The most important aspect of this issue, however, is that if we consider whether the project of cultured meat is morally sound by considering only sustainability and reduction of suffering, we might miss a lot of the ethical issues involved here. Under these guises, it would seem more appropriate to move toward an animal-free diet altogether rather than perpetrate meat eating. Still, if lab meat one day becomes readily available and affordable, and it tastes exactly like its authentic counterpart, what would be the moral problem at that point? As mentioned earlier, many meat eaters, arguably, would accept eating lab-grown meat. But what about vegans? It seems that vegans would have to accept growing meat in a lab as morally viable, which would be a very strange form of veganism. In my view, what could still be said against lab meat is its unvirtuous motivation. Namely, why are we as humans even contemplating eating food that is produced in a lab given the abundance of naturally grown plant-based food? The enterprise of creating meat in a laboratory seems obstinate and evinces a lack of temperance and a misunderstanding of the role of food. As humans, are we supposed to place so much importance on a food that we are willing to create it in a lab? Artificial meat production could arguably benefit the environment, but does this mean that lab-grown meat is likely to replace "real" meat? It seems to me that the idea of cultured meat is just another shrewd strategy to introduce yet another product into an already saturated market. The introduction of lab-grown meat might just become an option for the meat eater. "Which steak, sir? Lab-grown or farm-grown?" In the end it might make little to no difference to the current state of animals being raised for food.

It seems to me that there is something fundamentally wrong with the whole idea of cultured meat. At the risk of committing a false analogy, consider this comparison. The enterprise of producing meat in a lab seems to me like trying to find a way to reinstate slavery by studying the way to make it moral. But why even bother? If a practice is immoral, the lesson should be to avoid it altogether. Of course, my analogy implies that eating meat is immoral before proving that it is. However, the point here is not to try to show that this is the case. Rather, I want to show that the morality of eating meat, like that of slavery, should be understood with reference to good moral character rather than deontic or consequentialist values.

Consequentialists, it seems, would say that slavery is immoral because it is not conducive to maximum utility; deontology would say that slavery is immoral because it offends humanity or it violates human rights. In my view, slavery is immoral because it is an expression of vice. Or, to put it another way, a virtuous individual would not enslave or participate in or support the institution of slavery because it is the very antithesis of compassion and justice. Similarly, eating meat is immoral when it is done for trivial reasons, such as taste or tradition.

Virtue ethics, therefore, can make sense of this issue in a way that other theories can't because it does not stop at the consideration of what is most convenient. A virtue-based approach considers the motivation and character of an individual who would support the creation of lab-grown meat. What are the virtues and how can they help? Temperance in particular can make us see what is wrong with cultured meat. If we judge from the perspective of virtue, we realize that the issue of cloned meat is not merely of a practical nature. In a well-known article,[3] Anscombe pointed out that we should drop the idea of obligation altogether. And that is what we need to do if we wish to understand the morality of lab-grown meat. The current discussion is focused on the rightness or wrongness of such an endeavor. But all along there is an important question standing on the side, the question of our approach to the issue as good and rational individuals. Virtue ethics has the advantage of making sense of this issue by shifting the focus of the discussion to the character of the individual. Hence, it shows that a better approach to eating is one according to virtue. The pertinent virtue is temperance because, as Aristotle pointed out, temperance has to do with appetites, in the sense of physical or brutish appetites, as he put it in the *Ethics*. A temperate individual is one whose approach to eating is measured. As I hope it will emerge from this discussion, the idea of growing meat in laboratories evinces lack of temperance; consequently, in this sense I believe that ethical vegans should address the prospect of lab-grown meat as morally defective.

ETHICAL VEGANISM AND LAB-GROWN MEAT

Ethical veganism is the idea of avoiding consumption of animals and animal by-products to the best of our ability and whenever possible. It is, most importantly, a mark of virtue. Animal ethics has been dominated by deontology and consequentialism but should be approached instead from the perspective of a virtue-oriented ethics. Deontologists and consequentialists focus on moral rules or best outcomes and in so doing neglect the moral character of individuals, which is what I find to be the important aspect of morality. It seems to me peculiar that the discussion of our treatment of animals stems from a consideration of the kinds of rights animals might have or the way in which animals may or may not contribute to aggregate happiness. I suggest that being or becoming a vegan should be a moral decision based on the proper acquisition of certain important moral virtues, such as temperance, compassion, and greatness of soul. These and other virtues enable one to see animals in a different light, as individuals whose lives are important in their own right, and not as mere things that can be turned into food. Using the body parts or secretions of animals is common practice nowadays. But I suggest that by looking at the issue from the point of view of virtue, we might be able to understand the callousness of using animals for food.

A question that has always presented itself to vegans is this: "If meat could be grown in a lab without harming animals, would it be moral to produce it and consume it? Would vegans finally be content? What could they possibly complain about?" Vegans seem to be unready to address these questions. It seems that there can be ethical vegans on both sides of the debate. On the one hand, lab-grown meat could be the solution to the negative environmental impact of animal agriculture; moreover it may reduce or possibly end animal suffering. Some of the comments by people on vegetarian forums are very telling: "I hope that lab meat someday catches on and can help end animal suffering. However, I would probably gag," writes one user.[4] Another user writes, "I'm a vegetarian because of cruelty of factory farming and because of the terrible environmental impact it causes, so yes, I would eat the meat."[5] The issue of whether lab-grown meat is moral seems to be addressed in terms of taste, concern for the environment, and animal suffering that can be caused by animal farming. Taste does not seem to be important enough to justify animal exploitation, though as we will see it is a vital aspect that will determine meat eaters' acceptance of lab-made meat. However, environmental concern and animal suffering are very serious issues. In 2013, Dr. Mark Post's laboratory at Maastricht University in the Netherlands produced the first lab-grown burger. Dr. Post argued that growing meat in labs could reduce the impact of livestock production on the environment.[6] If this were the case, from an ethical point of view, it would seem that even the staunchest ethical vegans (like myself, for example), who detest the idea of eating meat regardless of its origin, would have nothing to object about it.

However, the morality of lab-grown meat is not as simple a question as it might appear.

I will discuss some of the positive and negative aspects of the issue and will later explore the possibility that considering lab-grown meat is a moral mistake that we might be able to see by embracing a virtue-oriented ethics.

There are several advantages to creating meat in a laboratory, the most evident of which is a smaller number of raised and killed animals. But it is not only a matter of reducing animal suffering. Fewer animals brought into existence and raised for consumption means a less severe impact upon the environment. Unfortunately, animal agriculture contributes to 51 percent of global greenhouse gas emissions,[7] using a third of the earth's fresh water, 45 percent of the Earth's land, causing 91 percent of Amazon rainforest destruction, and serving as a leading cause of species extinction, ocean dead zones, and habitat destruction.[8]

The good news about artificially grown meat, according to a 2011 study, is that "cultured meat involves approximately 7–45 percent lower energy use ... 78–96 percent lower GHG emissions, 99 percent lower land use, and 82–96 percent lower water use depending on the product compared."[9] These numbers sound great, just what an environmentalist wants to hear; however, they are theoretical since lab-grown meat is not yet a reality.

At this juncture, the reality of cultured meat is unknown, and so is its actual environmental impact, though it seems reasonable to say that under ideal conditions, all things being equal, meat grown in the lab could be a more sustainable reality than the current practice of animal farming.

Returning to the question of taste, as mentioned earlier, it is not a morally important aspect, though it is the aspect in which meat eaters are interested. One interesting point about cultured meat[10] is that the meat grown for the (in)famous 2013 burger experiment was not exactly ideal by meat eaters' standards. The meat produced by Dr. Post in his lab was merely lean muscle fibers. It lacked the typical characteristics of meat, such as fat, nerves, and blood, which are the very elements that give meat its characteristic taste and texture. In order to create something that resembles the "real deal" in both taste and consistency, the muscle fiber has to be "exercised" and supplied with artificial blood flow, oxygen, and nutrition.[11] These achievements are no small potato. And though I personally doubt this will be possible, it is not excluded that the project could be actualized in the future. If, in the future, scientists will be capable of producing lab-made meat that is identical or nearly identical to real meat, then at that point consuming lab meat rather than "real" meat would contribute to reduction in land usage and energy usage—provided that meat eaters would have no issue consuming lab-grown meat, that is.[12] Another obvious factor is whether it would be possible to produce meat at a reasonable cost. But once again, at this juncture it is a bit premature to claim any environmental benefits.

Arguably one of the most desirable aspects of lab meat is that, if actualized, it would reduce the number of animals that are brought into existence, and thus reduce suffering. This is all well and good, of course. Proponents of cultured meat make exactly this point. I am the first in line when it comes to less suffering in the world. But then, as important as reducing suffering is, I don't believe suffering is the sole factor to be considered in determining the morality of lab-grown meat. This issue is typically addressed within the moral framework of consequentialist and deontic ethics (or some variation of these two). Considered from a consequentialist standpoint, the question of the morality of lab-grown meat would seem quite clear-cut. According to consequentialist ethics, an action is just if its consequences lead to the promotion of aggregate happiness and a reduction of the amount of overall suffering. Assuming that in the near future lab-meat scientists achieve their goal of producing meat that tastes the same as traditional meat, and they can produce it at an affordable cost, a consequentialist would certainly approve it. Under this assumption, animal suffering will be dramatically reduced or perhaps even eliminated while meat eaters would have their fix and be happy. This seems to be the perfect formula for a utilitarian. And that is the end of the story. Rights theorists or deontologists would differ in their approach, in the sense that the goal of deontology is to do the right thing for the right reason, but they also would have no problem supporting production of lab meat. As I shall discuss later, however, I suggest that the story does not end there if we consider it from the standpoint of a virtue-based approach. However, there are several factors to take into account before it can be said that lab-grown meat can reduce animal suffering. One of these issues is that to be cruelty-free, some might suggest, it should be animal-free. The challenge at present is for scientists to find a method of self-renewing stem cells and animal-free materials to accomplish growth. Namely, researchers are still working on the possibility of an initial harvesting of animal cells that in the long run will no longer require subsequent harvesting. Furthermore, researchers are looking for a suitable plant-based material that will serve as "scaffolding" for the development of animal cells into a hunk of meat.

Very roughly explained, cells are taken from a living animal and allowed to grow in a petri dish in a laboratory. In practical terms, the initial harvested cells are taken from animals that are raised according to specification so that their flesh can be genetically emulated in a lab. But is that the end of the process? Are animals off the hook after that (pun intended)? It seems not. Dr. Post points out that "the most efficient way of taking the process forward would still involve slaughter [using a] limited herd of donor animals."[13] In other words, assuming that lab-grown meat becomes a reality, it would still be necessary to raise animals and use them as cell banks, so to speak, for fresh cells to be harvested and grown artificially into flesh. Granted, the number of animals involved would be considerably smaller than the current number of raised and slaughtered animals, and suffering would be minimal to no suffering at all. It will not, however, dispense with the use of animals altogether. It is hard to imagine how it could ever be possible to produce meat in a lab without ever involving live animals. However, some argue that, eventually, it will be possible to establish a self-renewing stem cell line; that is, it will be possible to start the process by an initial biopsy and get it going without resorting to further harvesting.[14] If this were the case (and of course at this point it is just speculation), considering the wants of meat lovers and the astute operations of the market, meat eaters might see that the sky is the limit when it comes to variety and taste. I want to be very careful here not to suggest something that might be understood as a slippery-slope fallacy; but at that point, if growing meat becomes as easy as researchers hope it to be, why not clone any kind of animal meat, including, but not limited to, wild animals. And again, not trying to open the proverbial can of worms here, what would be a moral objection to lab-grown human meat? Obviously it would not be human meat because it would be a lab product, but nevertheless it could taste like human flesh and could be marketed as such. Labs would start harvesting cells from all kinds of animals (including, perhaps, human animals) or breeding exotic animals especially for cell harvesting, which would take us right back to square one and, once again, require breeding animals for food. Granted, it would involve an initial harvesting; but it seems that as the demand of variety increases, the number of initial harvesting processes will continue.

The next point, as mentioned, is an issue that is seldom addressed in the discussion of lab-grown meat. This issue is the type of support that would hold the lab-grown muscle. At present, bovine fetal serum, which is an animal by-product, is used. The harvesting of bovine fetal serum is, obviously, not ideal from a vegan standpoint. Typically, the serum is obtained by sticking a needle into the heart of a fetal cow.

> At the time of slaughter, the cow is found to be pregnant during evisceration (removal of the internal organs in the thorax and abdomen during processing

of the slaughtered cow).... The calf is removed quickly from the uterus [and] a cardiac puncture is performed by inserting a needle between the ribs directly into the heart of the unanaesthesised [*sic*] fetus and blood is extracted. This bleeding process can take up to 35 minutes to complete while the calf remains alive. Afterwards, the fetus is processed for animal feed and extraction of specific substances like fats and proteins, among other things.[15]

A study considers whether the cows can feel this procedure and the possibility of slow death from lack of oxygen due to placental separation; it also estimates that approximately two million fetuses are harvested annually for serum.[16] If the point of growing meat is to reduce suffering, then fetal serum does not seem to be the way to go. For that reason, scientists are already working hard to find plant-based alternatives.[17]

From a very practical point of view, perhaps from a consequentialist standpoint, all this hard work and dedication to cultured meat that is identical to real meat, and the work dedicated to finding a replacement to fetal serum with a suitable plant-based alternative, seems normal. After all, ingenuity is one of the primary characteristics of humanity. Every obstacle is there for us to overcome. We put men on the moon, and very soon on Mars, so growing ethical meat in a lab seems like just the next challenge. Though I think there is something almost perverse about the motivation and tenacity of scientists in making lab-grown meat a reality, I will refrain from saying anything at this juncture. I will, instead, consider another aspect of this issue that could be considered positive. Recent literature has provided some substantial evidence that consumption of meat can cause a variety of health issues. The good news (such as it is) is that the supposed lab-made meat can potentially be manipulated to avoid the leading causes of health conditions. The FDA said in a statement, "Given information we have at the time, it seems reasonable to think that cultured meat, if manufactured in accordance with appropriate safety standards and all relevant regulations, could be consumed safely."[18] Other studies argue that since meat is literally grown in a laboratory by scientists, it could be possible to decide the amount and type of fat cells and other dietary characteristics of the final product. Furthermore, since slaughtering would no longer be necessary, the threat of pathogens and contamination would be reduced or eliminated.[19] I think the obvious question is "How would the FDA or any other possibly know?" I am not suggesting that we should not trust scientific data—if that is indeed what we have at hand. But once again, we have no idea what long-term effects artificial meat might have on health.

To add one more "if" to the list, provided that scientists will eventually be able to grow meat without harvesting cells from living animals, find a plant-based growth medium, reduce or eliminate animal suffering, and reduce the damage caused by animal farming, should we not abandon our moral reservations about lab-grown meat? One obvious issue can be put thus: Who would want to eat meat that was grown in a laboratory? Surveys seem to suggest that the majority of people would be, to put it candidly, very reluctant to ingest lab-grown meat.[20] Granted, proponents of cultured meat remind us that "lab-grown" is a misleading term. That is to say, at present, for obvious reasons, research is being conducted in laboratories; but eventually, the meat would be made in factories. As Mattick and Allenby point out, "A world where meat comes mostly from factories instead of ranches and feedlots might be a world better able to deal with challenges of food security, the environment, and natural resources."[21] In fact, growing meat could provide a reliable and safe way to make sure that meat is devoid of hormones, antibiotics, and other chemicals that typically are given to animals.

However, some commentators still remain unconvinced. The CEO of SAFE makes a valid point:

> It is also possible that in order to overcome the public resistance to [lab-grown meat] governments and charities will be asked to fund PR campaigns and meet the research and development costs of [lab meat]. This could possibly lead to public revenue being spent on developing and promoting a technology and product that the majority of the public do not want and that will be of benefit to only those who can afford it. The Dutch government has already funded research into [lab-grown meat] conducted by New Harvest.[22]

But it might be objected that even so, funding research is justified because it will be for the benefit of the environment and the animals. After all, the argument might go, at this point it does not seem likely to hope for a vegan world. People do not seem to be interested in avoiding animal products. So rather than fighting the current issue of animal exploitation, which seems to be an uphill battle, we ought to search for practical and viable solutions to replace meat—and the solution is lab-grown meat.[23] After all, that is exactly the supposed function of the various mock meats on the market. Nowadays stores carry all kinds of plant-based mock versions of meats and even cheese. The manufacturers as well as the consumers of those products point out that such products are environmentally safe. Thus, lab-grown meat should be viewed as mock meat—the best possible mock meat because it is exactly like meat (assuming, of course that scientist are able to create a perfect replica). An organization called Why Cultured Meat, for example, argues that lab-grown meat can do more for the benefit of animals and the environment than ethical veganism could ever dream of. They argue that providing an alternative that not only looks and tastes like meat, like Tofurkey or vegan meatballs, but actually is meat, could be (again, assuming that lab-meat researchers are successful) the most effective and viable path to the desired "animal liberation." If actualized, production of lab-grown meat could mean the abolition of factory farms and hence the avoidance of suffering for millions of animals. Furthermore, if everything goes according to plan, production and consumption of lab-grown meat could mean a healthier environment.

At that point, what would be (if any) the objections of vegans to cultured meat? In the best-case scenario, assume that researchers in the future will achieve a lab meat that is a perfect replica of real meat in taste and everything else, and as a result animals and the environment will benefit from it. Shouldn't vegans and animal rights activists be happy? After all, those who avoid animal-based products for ethical reasons argue that it is immoral to eat meat because it causes animal suffering and affects the environment in a negative way. I think the answers to these and similar questions are predicated upon the kind of idea one assumes about morality. In other words, it depends on the moral outlook from which the issue of cultured meat is considered. As Anscombe points out in her frequently cited article, "Modern Moral Philosophy," ethics typically assumes the notion of obligation or moral ought. She writes, "It would be a great improvement if, instead of 'morally wrong,' one always named a genus such as 'untruthful,' 'unchaste,' 'unjust.'"[24] The important message of Anscombe and many others who think about morality is that moral problems require the kind of approach that a virtue-based theory can offer. It seems to me that the question of the morality of producing and consuming cultured meat is typically dealt with by a consideration of our duty or consideration of rights. Robert B. Louden, referring to Anscombe's remark, writes, "But are we to take the assertion literally, and actually attempt to do moral theory without any concept of duty?"[25] As far as I understand Anscombe, I do not think that she meant that we should do away with duty altogether. Perhaps I am wrong about what Anscombe really believed, but I am not suggesting here that duty is an unimportant aspect in morality. Rather, I want to suggest that in many cases trying to figure out our duty leads us nowhere. In the present issue, what is our duty? Ought we not to be saving the world from environmental degradation? Or ought we not to avoid injustice and gratuitous suffering? The answer obviously seems to be "yes." And if lab-grown meat is capable of doing that, then we have a duty to support lab-grown meat; consequently, according to duty ethics, that's the end of the story. But I think that a virtue-oriented approach is the correct framework to make sense of this issue, because an ethics of virtue enables us to see aspects of moral issues that are simply discounted by other moral theories.

ABORTION AND MEAT

To see why the moral viability of lab-grown meat requires the attention of virtue ethics, I want to discuss the famous article "Virtue Theory and Abortion," by Rosalind Hursthouse, where she discusses the morality of abortion in a way that parallels my argument here: "The abortion is commonly discussed in relation to just two considerations: first . . . the status of the fetus . . . ; secondly . . . women's rights. . . . Virtue theory quite transforms the discussion of abortion by dismissing the two familiar dominating considerations as, in a way, fundamentally irrelevant."[26] And it seems to me that the question of the morality of cultured meat is often approached in relation to our duty and to the best consequences. No reference is ever made to virtue and character. Hursthouse's argument is that considering an issue such as abortion in the light of rights or duty is not helpful at all. In the case of abortion, questions of the status of the fetus and of women's rights are two of the most complicated questions in morality. The status of the fetus is a very controversial issue that may never be settled. And how far should the rights of women go is not a straightforward issue either. The advantage of virtue theory is to view the issue of abortion in a broader perspective by primarily considering, among other things, one's character. VE asks whether or not a certain action is in accordance with certain admirable traits of one's character. Because every situation is different, it is often very hard to be able to figure out what our duty is. A woman's pregnancy could be the result of accident, rape, or love. Consequently, whether abortion is right or not depends on the nature of that specific case.

Hursthouse makes clear that her analysis of the morality of abortion is distinct from a question about whether women "have a moral right to terminate their pregnancies" precisely because "in exercising a moral right I can do something cruel, or callous, or selfish, light-minded, self-righteous, stupid, inconsiderate, disloyal, dishonest—that is, act viciously."[27] Regarding the status of the fetus, she claims that "it is a metaphysical question," and therefore it is unreasonable to expect to come to a conclusion and use it as grounds for proper moral analysis of abortion. VE does not attempt to answer metaphysical questions of that nature, but rather tries to analyze morality with the resources at hand. The reason for this is that "the sort of knowledge that the fully virtuous person has is not supposed to be recondite."[28] In other words, since the virtuous person should be able to make moral judgments on the basis of reason and common knowledge, it cannot be the case that moral judgment about abortion would have to hinge on an impervious metaphysical question. Reasonable judgment, Hursthouse notes, ought to be made on the basis of "familiar biological facts," which are "the facts that most human societies are and have been familiar with."[29]

Hursthouse then gives examples of the kind of facts she has in mind: "standardly (but not invariably), pregnancy occurs as the result of sexual intercourse, that it lasts about nine months, during which time the fetus grows and develops, that standardly it terminates in the birth of a living baby, and that this is how we all come to be."[30]

Considering these facts, then, Hursthouse suggests the question should be, "How do these familiar biological facts figure in the practical reasoning, actions and passions, thoughts and reactions, of the virtuous and the non-virtuous? What is the mark to having the right attitude to these facts and what manifests having the wrong attitude to them?"[31] Her starting point is to note that abortion is a serious matter because it concerns "in some sense, the cutting off of a new human life." To dismiss it forthright reflects a fundamental misunderstanding of what is at stake. Accordingly, "to think of abortion as nothing but the killing of something that does not matter, or as nothing but the exercise of some right . . . or as the incidental means to some desirable state of affairs, is to do something callous and light-minded, the sort of thing that no virtuous and wise person would do."[32] Deontological and utilitarian approaches, Hursthouse points out, are inadequate to appreciating the seriousness of life and of what is at stake in abortion.

VE realizes that abortion is an intrinsically important matter because "by virtue of the fact that a human life has been cut short, some evil has probably been brought about."[33] It does not mean, however, that abortion is *categorically* wrong. Rather a choice in favor of an abortion in a particular case must be weighed in light of the relevant virtues and in light of the way that abortion might or might not be conducive to a good life. In other words, it is necessary to take into account and weigh certain goods, such as the value of the human life that is cut off with abortion, the value of motherhood/parenthood for a woman, and their contribution toward living a good, noble human life. Therefore, in order to be valid, a choice for abortion in a particular case must be granted by a desire to obtain or preserve goods that are superior to those goods that abortion cuts off.

VE thus is not about generating "some general rule such as 'You ought not to kill anything with a right to life but may kill anything else.'"[34] However, at the same time it is the best approach to abortion because it includes in the discussion important factors and particularities of specific contexts and circumstances that other theories wrongly discount. It is seldom possible, and certainly not desirable, to derive some abstract principle that will always allow us to accurately discriminate between legitimate abortions and those that are not. Rather, abortion is best understood by approaching each case individually and asking whether in a particular case the goods being pursued are commensurate with the ones that abortion cuts off.

Hursthouse gives several examples of justified abortions: a mother of several children who "fears that to have another will seriously affect her capacity to be a good mother to the ones she has," "a woman who has been a good mother and is approaching the age at which she may be looking forward to being a good grandmother," "a woman who discovers that her pregnancy may well kill her," or even "a woman who has decided to lead a life centered around some other worthwhile activity or activities with which motherhood would compete."[35] She also gives examples of women in positions that are so unfortunate that a decision in favor of abortion is the "right" one: "To go through a pregnancy when one is utterly exhausted, or when one's job consists of crawling along tunnels hauling coal . . . is perhaps heroic, but people who do not achieve heroism are not necessarily vicious."[36] However, Hursthouse points out that "this does not make everything all right . . . it shows that there is something amiss with the conditions of [these women's] lives, which are making it impossible for them to live well."[37] Such women have an unfortunate life and, though it is a disgraceful event, abortion perhaps is a way to ameliorate their lives. An abortion in such cases can be morally justified when a woman still manifests "the right attitude to human life and death."

Hursthouse contrasts the right attitude with that of women who choose abortion for "worthless" ends such as "having a good time" or for "the pursuit of some false vision of the ideals of freedom or self-realization." She argues against those motivated by an unreasonable dream "of having two perfect children, a girl and a boy, within a perfect marriage, in financially secure circumstances, with an interesting job of one's own."[38] Choosing abortion in pursuit of an unrealistic life or a false vision of the good is vicious. Consequently, considering the issue of abortion from the point of view of VE, Hursthouse makes seemingly radical claims that the status of the fetus and the issue of women's rights are "in a way, fundamentally irrelevant." According to VE, the central issue in evaluating whether or not abortion is permissible is essentially a question of whether or not a woman exhibits a virtuous or vicious character, whether or not a woman understands the nature of the real goods that abortion generally cuts off. If one is knowingly sacrificing these goods in order to follow "other worthwhile pursuits" conducive to flourishing, which are incompatible with having a child, or because a pregnancy would place excessive burdens on her (especially in light of a woman's health issue), she is not thereby manifesting a vicious character, and therefore her choice of abortion may be justified.

Critics often complain that VE is vague. But the reason for this sort of complaint is that VE does not offer any algorithm to calculate the proper course of action. It does not offer maximizing calculation as in utilitarianism or absolute moral rules as in deontology. I do not see these as criticisms but rather as attractive features of a moral theory. After all, in the case of abortion, since it is largely a woman's decision, what notions does a woman have other than her specific circumstances and her pursuit of a good life? Considering that it is possible to have an account of consistent, morally desirable virtues, a woman can correctly choose an abortion insofar as she acts in accordance with such virtues, provided she recognizes the value of the human life that is potentially cut off by abortion. Those goods described by Hursthouse are concrete factors and thus are not vague. Parenthood and motherhood contribute greatly to flourishing. Other approaches rely on the recondite metaphysical question of the status of the fetus or the difficult notion of competing rights.

But what can be learned from Hursthouse's discussion of the morality of abortion that is valuable to the question of the morality of cultured meat? I believe that when we approach this question with an attitude similar to that proposed by Hursthouse, we are immediately prompted to view the issue of cultured meat from a completely new angle; and we may realize that this new view features important issues that we have not yet contemplated. There are several points to be made.

It is no longer a mystery that factory-farmed animals suffer. But why do they suffer? They suffer because they are deprived of what makes them flourish: sunlight, freedom, their natural food, their families, and more. Factory farms are squalid places where animals are often crammed into cages so small that they cannot even move around. In addition to the lack of adequate space, animals live and defecate in the same quarters, they are given all kinds of supplements and hormones to prevent diseases, and they grow disproportionately big. The end is always the same—death followed by the flesh being cut up, packaged, and shipped to supermarkets. One of the reasons for this is that if the animals were allowed to live adequate lives, the cost of meat would be very high and the supply very low. Thus, the possibility of replacing factory-farmed animals with meat that cannot suffer seems enticing.

But if the concern is the "plight of animals," it seems that what is in play here is a virtuous attitude that is not yet brought to fruition. If the very project of cultured meat is justified in terms of reduction of suffering, it is clear that the idea behind it is that suffering is not okay—that is, that there is something inherently callous about allowing animals to suffer. Consequently, it would seem that the best solution would be consistentcy in the application of compassion, making a serious effort to do away with factory farming altogether, and educating the public and weening them out of animal products.

If the underlying concern is animal suffering, it just seems callous, greedy, and self-indulgent to eat meat in the first place. Meat is not a requirement for good health—in fact, quite to the contrary, science shows that animal products can be harmful to human health;[39] and considering that taste can easily be adjusted to plant food, rather than perpetuating the idea of meat, our efforts as a civilization should be toward pursuing ways to move toward a plant-based diet. Is it possible that we have made such a mess of things in the world by bringing into existence millions of animals for food—resulting in the irreversible degradation of the environment and of our health—that we now are contemplating eating lab-made food? It seems to me that cloning meat is just another step toward alienation from nature. As Bhat, Kumar, and Fayaz point out,

> Another problem with the in vitro meat production system is that it may alienate us from nature and animals and can be a step in our retreat from nature to live in cities. Cultured meat fits in with an increasing dependence on technology, and the worry is that this comes with an ever greater estrangement from nature. In the absence of livestock based farming, fewer areas of land will be affected by human activities which is good for nature but it may at the same time alienate us from nature.[40]

I think we can and should do better that that. VE can contribute to the discussion of cultured meat by pointing out that the enthusiasm about lab-grown meat is mostly due to self-indulgence (as well as short-sightedness). We should ask ourselves whether the mere taste of a food is so important that we are willing to produce it in a laboratory.

What I am referring to above is something along the lines of temperance, or lack thereof. The virtue of temperance can be understood as Aristotle noted by its connection with animality. For Aristotle, human beings are animals endowed with reason. As animals, they are naturally subject to appetites for food, drink, sex, and more. They are sensitive to the pleasures that the satisfaction of such appetites can bring. Since our animality is not the distinguishing aspect of our humanity, physical pleasures should not be of major importance to us. However, humans are susceptible to these pleasures because our animality is part of their essence. In other words, insofar as we are part animal and part rational being, we have to deal with all kinds of physical pleasures in a way that harmonizes with reason. This characterization seems to me a valuable insight because it is a practical observation that can be made independently of the Aristotelian account of it.

Temperate people relate properly to their animality and give the proper worth to animalistic pleasures. Insensible people and self-indulgent or intemperate people, in their respective way, misjudge the importance of certain pleasures and misjudge themselves. Intemperate people place too much importance on the pleasures of food and drink. We eat and drink primarily because we require nourishment. Thanks to the ease of modern civilization, people who live in affluent societies, in my view, have lost sight of this and have placed too much importance on food. Food nowadays, for those of us who live comfortably, is more than fuel for the body.

Food is necessary and pleasurable. But humans can (and indeed do) have the wrong desire for it; generally in affluent societies this is manifested by the excess of food that people eat. For example, according to the Office of Disease Prevention and Health Promotion's dietary guidelines for 2015 to 2020, "The typical eating patterns currently consumed by many in the United States do not align with the Dietary Guidelines."[41] To say that eating patterns in the United States "do not align with the dietary guidelines" is a very mild way to put it when we consider that "about three-fourths of the population" consumes a low amount of fruit and vegetables. Also, "more than half of the population is meeting or exceeding total grain and total protein foods recommendations, [and] are not meeting the recommendations for the subgroups within each of these food groups." In particular, "most Americans exceed the recommendations for added sugars, and saturated fats."[42] And saturated fats come mainly from animal sources, including meat and dairy products. Furthermore, "the eating patterns of many are too high in calories. . . . The high percentage of the population that is overweight or obese suggests that many in the United States overconsume calories . . . more than two-thirds of all adults and nearly one-third of all children and youth in the United States are either overweight or obese."[43] These facts, in my view, clearly show that something about our relation with food has gone completely wrong. These facts are not surprising considering that the idea of food, for many reasons and by many factors, has been distorted.

It seems clear that it is the lack of temperance that makes humans take pleasure in the wrong food and in the wrong way. Furthermore, self-indulgence leads to pain, more than it is required, when certain foods are missed. The self-indulgent person values food too highly, choosing it at the cost of health. Thus, in relation to the bodily pleasure of food, one can be either self-indulgent, weak-willed, self-controlled, temperate, or insensible. The temperate person will choose what is pleasant and conducive to health, which is in its turn conducive to flourishing. Consequently, since strong desires for food can easily lead us astray in terms of health, the temperate person desires simple food and in moderation. When we survey the health sciences, it is clear that the only foods that can lower and prevent many health problems are fruits and vegetables.[44] In fact, as far as I have researched, I have never seen any study, or heard any medical professional, warn us of eating fruit and vegetables with caution.

Synthesizing meat opens the door to the varieties of meat that can be produced. It seems plausible that if laboratories crack the code and succeed in creating perfect replicas of meats, the next step will very likely be replicating the flesh of endangered species, wild animals, and humans. Cannibalism is not a desirable practice in modern society, not only because the very idea of it is repulsive, but because it can also cause a disease known as Kuru.[45] But what if human flesh can be replicated without the risk of any disease? Though human flesh is unlikely to become a popular dish, given the curiosity of human beings, there is still the prospect of cloning it for human consumption. This may sound like a slippery-slope objection to lab-grown meat, but I don't think that it is in this case. I do not intend to pursue this as an argument against lab-grown meat but rather use the discussion to illustrate the kind of irrational path to which cloning meat leads.

Owen Schaefer and Julian Savulescu point out that

> The most obvious reaction to this possibility of human [in vitro meat] is to ban it. Just as, for instance, cloning is banned in the 13 US states and the European Union for moral reasons, we could put in place strict restrictions on the synthesis of human flesh for the purpose of consumption. Given common revulsion at the prospect of cannibalism, this reaction is indeed rather likely. However, it is too quick—we should ask first, what is so wrong with cannibalism of artificially created human cells and tissue that it must be banned?[46]

Here they point out that despite our gut feeling that cannibalism is wrong, in the end there is no good argument against eating human flesh as it merely amounts to a feeling of disgust. In fact, cannibalism is morally objectionable because it (typically but not always) involves killing a person and the desecration of a corpse. But if human flesh is cloned, then there is no killing or desecration involved. To produce in vitro human flesh for human consumption, harvesting cells from people who are willing to donate their cells would be required. In fact, this process may even become lucrative for people who might be paid for their cells. At that point, then, what would be wrong with eating human flesh?

Could it be disrespect toward humanity? Since there are no human beings required in the production of hypothetical in vitro human flesh, no disrespect could be done. Schaefer and Savulescu thus conclude that if we are worried about in vitro meat because of cannibalism, we should not worry at all, because such meat will be free of cruelty and disrespect. Therefore, the objections that are typically raised against lab-grown meat rely on violation of respect and disgust, but they are not strong enough to reject the project of cloning meat for human consumption. Fewer animals being slaughtered, fewer animals suffering, less pollution, and many other advantages, in their view, are powerful enough to show that we should support research into cultured meat.

Many opinions about cloned meat are similar to that of Schaefer and Savulescu. Namely, as already pointed out, it seems that there is a prevailing view about the moral viability of making lab-grown meat that hinges on broadly consequentialist and deontic principles. Virtue ethics is not necessarily against the best consequences or the notion of rights. However, those should not be the only aspects that matter. As we have seen in the discussion of Hursthouse about abortion, sometimes in the name of the best consequences or in the name of our rights, we might act in ways that are callous, self-indulgent, selfish, and so on. Thus, it would certainly be an admirable thing to reduce suffering and care for the environment. But is cloning meat the right way to accomplish those things? I would like to suggest what a virtue-oriented approach can add to the discussion, and in so doing I will address cannibalism in particular, though the larger scope is to address in vitro meat. What I would like to suggest is something along the lines of what Leon Kass refers to as "the wisdom of repugnance," which is the same concept that Midgley and others call the "yuck factor." This is the notion that a strong, negative reaction of disgust to a practice is in fact good enough evidence that such a practice is not morally sound or that there is something intrinsically wrong with it. Granted, this sounds just like an appeal to emotion fallacy. The appeal to emotion fallacy, we must remember, is an informal fallacy, which means that it is possible for the conclusion of an argument based on such premises to be true. Martha Nussbaum points out that the "yuck factor" or disgust has been used in many arguments throughout history as a justification for evil practices and institutions, such as slavery, torture, antisemitism, gender and sexual discrimination, and so on.[47] But it seems to me, and many others, that just because a feeling of disgust may lead to the wrong conclusion, it does not follow that this feeling should be discounted forthright. Our feeling of revulsion may not be in itself an argument against a practice, but it certainly signals that something requires our attention because it might be morally wrong. Surely we can in many cases supply reason to this feeling and construct an argument. But even in the case that a fully articulated argument is not forthcoming, I don't think that in certain cases one is not entitled to reject a practice—in this case in vitro meat—on the basis of disgust. In fact, Leon Kass seems to think so in his argument about the feeling of revulsion:

> Revulsion is not an argument; and some of yesterday's repugnances are today calmly accepted—though, one must add, not always for the better. In crucial cases, however, repugnance is the emotional expression of deep wisdom, beyond reason's power fully to articulate it. Can anyone really give an argument fully adequate to the horror which is father-daughter incest (even with consent), or having sex with animals, or mutilating a corpse, or eating human flesh, or even just (just!) raping or murdering another human being? Would anybody's failure to give full rational justification for his or her revulsion at these practices make that revulsion ethically suspect? Not at all. On the contrary, we are suspicious of those who think that they can rationalize away our horror, say, by trying to explain the enormity of incest with arguments only about the genetic risks of inbreeding.[48]

The natural feeling of repugnance at cannibalism, and in general at cultured meat, belongs in this category. We are repelled by the prospect of cannibalism and cloned meat because we feel directly that such a practice violates our moral virtues. What kind of person am I to support artificial meat when I thrive by eating plants and fruit? Is the taste of meat so important that we are willing to allow technology to take over our lives? These are some of the questions that are part of that feeling of disgust. Repugnance, thus, is a natural reaction against the excesses of human willfulness to distance itself from nature. In this case, I believe, the repugnance expressed at the prospect of producing meat artificially is justified. In the case of sexism, racism, slavery, and more, repugnance stems from contempt, anger, and self-delusion. Thus, nurturing and following that feeling is wrong. But in the case of cultured meat, repugnance is the outcry of our human nature that is being overtaken and changed by technology, the blind hunger for innovation, profit, and self-indulgence.

As a concluding remark, I would like to point out that my discussion about the morality of producing and eating lab-grown meat is supposed to illustrate what a virtue-oriented theory can add to the discussion. Moreover, it is a view that the ethical vegan might take with respect to the morality of in vitro meat. Ethical veganism, as I understand it, is the rejection of meat as food, whether it is from an animal or a lab. What I argue is that ethical veganism should be based on virtue rather than deontic or consequentialist principles.[49] Ethical veganism should be the embodiment of virtue and thus should reject the notion of using animals for our taste and pleasure because doing so evinces a lack of temperance, compassion, fairness, and magnanimity. Consequently, an ethical vegan should not support the production of any kind of meat. However, not all vegans think this way. For example, Ingrid Newkirk, founder and president of People for the Ethical Treatment of Animals (PETA), offered $1 million for successful production of lab-grown meat.[50] As an ethical vegan, this seems to me a peculiar form of veganism. In my view, the reason for this schism among vegans is the fact that the question of the morality of lab-grown meat has been framed typically in terms of potential future gains, which seems to me to be an approach of consequentialist nature; another typical approach is of deontic nature. These approaches seek to rationalize the question of lab-grown meat, and certainly in their way they seem to achieve the goal of demonstrating that cloning meat for human consumption is morally viable and makes a lot of sense to support the project. After all, isn't less pollution and less animal suffering what we all want?

Yes, but as I hope to have shown, while those are important factors, they are not the only factors to be considered. Focusing only on those factors may lead to a tunnel-vision understanding of the issue. The contribution of a virtue-oriented approach is to show that, for example, the way we are going about reducing suffering and environmental degradation seems to completely disregard the importance of having an admirable character. In a recent article, Jean-François Hocquette aptly concluded that "the global scientific community including the proponents of artificial meat themselves recognize the hurdles to overcome so that artificial meat can progress to the industrial stage (new formulation of culture media, development of giant incubators, safety assessment for human consumption, etc.).[51] He also noted that there are other alternatives to cultured meat that are "faster to develop in the short term and more effective in responding to today's issues (in particular it is the case of the reduction of waste) compared to artificial meat which still needs a great deal of research."[52] A viable solution is, of course, that of plant-based meat substitutes, though in my view it would be more sustainable in the long run if we take steps toward abandoning what I regard as a primitive idea of animals as human food.

CONCLUSION

In light of the difficulties involved in the research for the production of viable in vitro meat, the virtue-based approach I suggest is to ask the following questions: Is meat so important for humans that we are willing to alienate ourselves from nature more and more by producing food in laboratories? Is meat so important that we are willing to continue the culture of carnism?[53] Is it so important that we must produce synthetic meat to "save" the environment and reduce animal cruelty and suffering when it would be much easier to adopt plant-based diets? My answer to these questions, of course, is no. Critics may, naturally, object to many of the points I made, but the overall point of my discussion has been that virtue theory has the resources to show why ethical veganism should not support in vitro meat; also, my aim was to show that moral issues are better understood when framed in terms of virtue and vice rather than in terms of best consequences or of rights.

NOTES

1. Gretchen Vogel, "Organs Made to Order," *Smithsonian Magazine*, August 2010, https://www.smithsonianmag.com/science-nature/organs-made-to-order-863675/.

2. Johns Hopkins Bloomberg School of Public Health, "Health and Environmental Implications of U.S. Meat Consumption & Production," https://www.jhsph.edu/research/centers-and-institutes/johns-hopkins-center-for-a-livable-future/projects/meatless_monday/resources/meat_consumption.html.

3. G. E. M. Anscombe, "Modern Moral Philosophy," *Philosophy* 33, no. 124 (1958): 1–19.

4. The_Einsteinian_God, "Would Meat Grown in a Lab Change Your Mind about Eating Meat?" *Reddit*, accessed August 23, 2018, https://www.reddit.com/user/the_einsteinian_god.

5. Ibid.

6. Arielle Duhaime-Ross, "Test-Tube Burger: Lab-Cultured Meat Passes Taste Test (Sort of)," *Scientific American*, August 5, 2013, https://www.scientificamerican.com/article/test-tube-burger-lab-culture/. See also, BBC News, "World's First Lab-Grown Burger Is Eaten in London," https://www.bbc.com/news/science-environment-23576143.

7. Robert Goodland and Jeff Anhang, "Livestock and Climate Change," Worldwatch Institute, http://www.worldwatch.org/node/6294.

8. The following is a list of sources: Mario Herrero et al., "Biomass Use, Production, Feed Efficiencies, and Greenhouse Gas Emissions from Global Livestock Systems," *Proceedings of the National Academy of Sciences* 110, no. 52 (December 24, 2013): 20888–93, doi:10.1073/pnas.1308149110; Richard Oppenlander, "Freshwater Abuse and Loss: Where Is It All Going?" *Forks over Knives*, May 20, 2013; Mesfin M. Mekonnen and Arjen Y. Hoekstra, "A Global Assessment of the Water Footprint of Farm Animal Products," *Ecosystems* 15, no. 3 (April 2012): 401–15, doi:10.1007/s10021-011-9517-8; P. W. Gerbens-Leenes, M. M. Mekonnen, and A. Y. Hoekstra, "The Water Footprint of Poultry, Pork and Beef: A Comparative Study in Different Countries and Production Systems," Water Resources and Industry, Water Footprint Assessment (WFA) for better water governance and sustainable development, 1–2

(March 2013): 25–36, doi:10.1016/j.wri.2013.03.001; Pete Smith, Bustamante Mercedes, et al., "Agriculture, Forestry and Other Land Use (AFOLU)"; Philip Thornton, Mario Herrero, and Polly Ericksen, "Livestock and Climate Change," International Livestock Research Institute 2011, cgspace.Cgiar.org/bitstream/handle/10568/10601/IssueBrief3. Pdf; Richard Oppenlander, *Food Choice and Sustainability: Why Buying Local, Eating Less Meat, and Taking Baby Steps Won't Work* (Minneapolis, MN: Langdon Street Press, 2013); Sérgio Margulis, "Causes of Deforestation of the Brazilian Amazon," World Bank Working Paper, no. 22 (2004); "Press Release Louisiana Universities Marine Consortium," August 4, 2014; "What Causes Ocean 'Dead Zones'?" *Scientific American*, February 27, 2016; Environmental Protection Agency, "What's the Problem? Animal Waste Region 9 US EPA," accessed February 27, 2016; Henning Steinfeld et al., "Livestock's Long Shadow"; World Wildlife Fund, "Impact of Habitat Loss on Species," accessed February 27, 2016; Center for Biological Diversity, "How Eating Meat Hurts Wildlife and the Planet: Take Extinction off Your Plate."

9. Hanna L. Tuomisto and M. Joost Teixeira de Mattos, "Environmental Impacts of Cultured Meat Production," *Environmental Science & Technology* 45, no. 14 (July 15, 2011): 6117–23, doi:10.1021/es200130u.

10. Henceforth, I will use the terms "lab-grown meat," "cultured meat," or other such equivalent terms interchangeably.

11. Alok Jha, "Synthetic Meat: How the World's Costliest Burger Made It on to the Plate," *The Guardian*, August 5, 2013; Nick Collins, "Test Tube Hamburgers to Be Served This Year," February 19, 2012; Carolyn S. Mattick et al., "Anticipatory Life Cycle Analysis of In Vitro Biomass Cultivation for Cultured Meat Production in the United States," *Environmental Science & Technology* 49, no. 19 (October 6, 2015): 11941–49, doi:10.1021/acs.est.5b01614; Carolyn Mattick et al., "The Problem with Making Meat in a Factory," *Slate*, September 28, 2015.

12. Ibid.

13. Nick Collins, "Test Tube Hamburgers to Be Served This Year," *The Telegraph*, February 19, 2012, https://www.telegraph.co.uk/news/science/science-news/9091628/Test-tube-hamburgers-to-be-served-this-year.html.

14. "Why Cultured Meat—FAQ," accessed March 25, 2016; "The Crusade for a Cultured Alternative to Animal Meat: An Interview with Nicholas Genovese, PhD PETA," accessed March 25, 2016; "New Harvest—FAQ," *New Harvest*, accessed March 26, 2016, http://whyculturedmeat.org/faq/.

15. Carlo E. A. Jochems et al., "The Use of Fetal Bovine Serum: Ethical or Scientific Problem?" ATLA-Nottingham 30, no. 2 (2002): 219–28.

16. Ibid.

17. Mirko Betti and Isah Datar, "Possibilities for an In Vitro Meat Production System," *Innovative Food Science & Emerging Technologies* 1 (2010): 13–22, doi:10.1016/j.ifset.2009.10.007.

18. Charlotte Hawks, "How Close Are We to a Hamburger Grown in a Lab?" CNN, https://www.cnn.com/2018/03/01/health/clean-in-vitro-meat-food/index.html.

19. M. Specter, "Test-Tube Burgers," *The New Yorker*, May 23, 2011, https://www.newyorker.com/magazine/2011/05/23/test-tube-burgers.

20. Diana Fleischman, "Lab Meat: Survey Results," *The Vegan Option Radio Show and Blog*, May 16, 2012; Vegetarian Society, "Vegetarian Society Quick Polls," accessed March 24, 2016; Wim Verbeke et al., "Would You Eat Cultured Meat? Consumers Reactions and Attitude Formation in Belgium, Portugal and the United Kingdom," *Meat Science* 102 (April 2015): 49–58, doi:10.1016/j.meatsci.2014.11.013; "YouGov No British Demand for Fake Meat," *YouGov: What the World Thinks*, accessed March 25, 2016; Daniel M. T. Fessler, Alexander P. Arguello, Jeannette M. Mekdara, and Ramon Macias, "Disgust Sensitivity and Meat Consumption: A Test of an Emotivist Account of Moral Vegetarianism," *Appetite* 41, no. 1 (August 2003): 31–41, doi:10.1016/S0195-6663(03)00037-0.

21. Carolyn Mattick and Brad Allenby, "The Future of Meat: Issues in Science and Technology," *Issues in Science and Technology* XXX, no. 1 (Fall 2013).

22. Jasmijn de Boo, "The Future of Food, Why Lab Grown Meat Is Not the Solution," *Huffpost*, September 8, 2013, https://www.huffingtonpost.co.uk/jasmijn-de-boo/lab-grown-meat_b_3730367.html.

23. See many arguments offered in favor of cultured meat by Why Cultured Meat, http://whyculturedmeat.org/essays/animal-rights/is-it-animal-rights/.

24. G. E. M. Anscombe, "Modern Moral Philosophy," *Philosophy* 33, no. 124 (1958): 1–19. Reprinted in J. J. Thompson and G. Dworkin, (eds.), *Ethics* (New York: Harper and Row, 1968), 89.

25. Louden, "On Some Vices of Virtue Ethics," *American Philosophical Quarterly* 21 (1984): 228.

26. Hursthouse, "Virtue Theory and Abortion," 233.

27. Ibid., 235.

28. Ibid., 235.

29. Ibid., 236.

30. Ibid., 236.

31. Ibid., 237.

32. Ibid., 237–38.

33. Ibid., 242.

34. Ibid., 236.

35. Ibid., 241–2.

36. Ibid., 239–40.

37. Ibid., 239–40.

38. Ibid., 242.

39. University of Southern California, "Meat and Cheese May Be as Bad for You as Smoking," *ScienceDaily*, www.sciencedaily.com/releases/2014/03/140304125639.htm (accessed June 20, 2018).

40. Zuhaib Fayaz Bhat, Sunil Kumar, and Hina Fayaz, "In Vitro Meat Production," *Journal of Integrative Agriculture* 14, no. 2 (February 2015): 246. https://doi.org/10.1016/S2095-3119(14)60887-X.

41. "Current Eating Patterns in the United States," *Dietary Guidelines 2015-2020* (2015), https://health.gov/dietaryguidelines/2015/guidelines/chapter-2/current-eating-patterns-in-the-united-states/.

42. Ibid.

43. Ibid.

44. Harvard T. H. Chan School of Public Health, "Vegetables and Fruits," https://www.hsph.harvard.edu/nutritionsource/what-should-you-eat/vegetables-and-fruits/.

45. Gajdusek DC, Zigas V., "Degenerative Disease of the Central Nervous System in New Guinea: The Endemic Occurrence of "Kuru" in the Native Population." *New Engl. J. Med.* 257 (1957): 974–978.

46. G. O. Schaefer and J. Savulescu, "The Ethics of Producing In Vitro Meat," *Journal of Applied Philosophy* 31, no. 2 (2014): 188–202, http://doi.org/10.1111/japp.12056.

47. M. Nussbaum, "Danger to Human Dignity," *The Chronicle of Higher Education* (2004).

48. Leon R. Kass, "The Wisdom of Repugnance," *The New Republic* 216, no. 22, June 2, 1997: 20.

49. Carlo Alvaro, "Ethical Veganism, Virtue, and Greatness of the Soul," *J. Agric. Environ. Ethics* 30 (2017): 765, https://doi.org/10.1007/s10806-017-9698-z; Carlo Alvaro, "Veganism as a Virtue: How Compassion and Fairness Show Us What Is Virtuous about Veganism," *Future of Food: Journal of Food, Agriculture and Society* 5, no. 2 (2017).

50. Ashley Phillips, "PETA Offers $1M Prize for Lab-Grown Meat," ABC News, April 23, 2008, https://abcnews.go.com/Technology/story?id=4704447&page=1.

51. J. F. Hocquette, "Is In Vitro Meat the Solution for the Future?" *Meat Sci.* 120 (October 2016):167–176, doi: 10.1016/j.meatsci.2016.04.036.

52. Ibid., 9.

53. See, Beyond Carnism, "What is Carnism?" https://www.carnism.org/carnism.

Conclusion

I once had a conversation with a person who was making a remark about the beauty of some dogs. He indicated that he liked dogs, and animals in general. Then, strangely, but not totally by accident, he began talking about food. When he mentioned to me a few of his favorite meat dishes, I explained to him that I do not eat meat. Bemused by my statement, he asked, "But what about fish?" So, I spelled it out for him: "Think about what fish is. It is a delicate and beautiful creature that schools with her friends. Eating fish means trapping that beautiful creature, destroying her life, and cutting her open with a knife. Cut open, that creature has blood, fluids, and guts coming out of her. How could I possibly eat that?" He looked at me for a moment before he replied, "Yeah, but you wash that"!

This funny episode (at least funny for me) came to my mind as I completed this work. One of the ideas that I have stressed in this book is that social and economic forces constantly try to educate us out of our virtues of compassion, fairness, temperance, and magnanimity; not surprisingly, it is usual in society that many people who love animals at the same time regard animals as food. This, I have argued, results from the disconnection between our moral feelings and our actions—that is, between our feelings toward animals and the food we eat. Some might call this moral schizophrenia, a case where one has genuine respect and love for animals but at the same time eats meat. The anecdote above is a good example of this.

It is very hard for people to shake the idea that animals are not our things that we can eat or wear or with which we stuff our pillows. But such an idea is not natural. It is an idea inculcated in us. At a very early age, we are exposed to a deceptive treatment that uses misleading language, behaviors, and images to condition us into believing that animals are our property and food. I believe that a viable animal ethics must focus on these issues first rather than trying to figure out the status of animals, their rights, or their utility. As I see it, a viable animal ethics must overcome two obstacles. The first one is that many people have been disciplined by moral systems—that is, deontology and utilitarianism. These are moral theories. I want to emphasize the word *theory* because these two systems have taught many thinkers that morality is something that can be captured by abstract concepts and calculi and turned into universal principles that can guide our actions. Such theories propose to do morality from the outside in, from external rules to behavior. The problem, however, is that when we theorize and use abstract rules, we detach ourselves from reality and we miss many important factors that allow us to make moral decisions, such as our relationship with others and their particular needs and values. Conversely, I have argued, morality is a social practice that requires virtuous character. Morality, in the view that I expressed here, needs to be done from the inside out. Namely, we must first worry about acquiring a good character—that is, a character that reflects the virtues. The trouble with theories such as utilitarianism, rights theory, and deontology is that they deal with humans and animals in a detached manner. Worse, they deny the importance of character, motivation, care, and relationship. Such theories lack the sort of attention to detail and to aspects of living with others that are necessary to move people to oppose animal exploitation. It is through the acquisition of virtue that we can see that humans and animals have genuine moral characteristics or value. The dominant theories in animal ethics, not surprisingly, are incapable of motivating us to respect animals. In other words, by focusing on common denominators such as sentience or rights, these theories strip off all the important differences that make humans and animals morally important.

Incidentally, these are the very moral theories that started the conversation and made us realize that we have moral obligations toward animals, whether we like it or not. For this I have an immense respect for Peter Singer and Tom Regan. The problem, however, is that their theories, and their variations, are based on invalid arguments, and thus are ineffective at convincing people to become vegans. The second obstacle has to do with deceiving language and other manipulative means that are deliberately used by the meat industry to hinder our acquisition of the virtues. Because of their financial interest, the meat industry, hunting, and scientific research adopt a deceiving, euphemistic language to hide the horror of animal exploitation that happens before our eyes and mislead us into believing that our treatment of animals is morally unproblematic. Thus, making real changes will also require another virtue that I hardly discussed, the virtue of courage. Policy makers will need the courage to make radical changes and implement policies that save the natural environment. This will involve the phasing out of animal-based industries; the replacement of animal-based food in schools; the introduction of moral education early on; showing through examples that animals and humans are already in a relationship, but the current relationship is not fair; and the teaching of morality as an expression of virtue.

My contribution to the discussion of our moral responsibility toward animals is to provide a consistent moral framework—a moral lifestyle, rather than a moral theory, that motivates us internally to become vegans. I proposed a view of morality according to which we acquire and develop important moral virtues, particularly the virtues of compassion, fairness, temperance, and greatness of soul, by paying attention to the lives of animals. Much work still needs to be done on the application of virtue/care ethics to eating with regard to our relationships with animals and with regard to the environment, public health, and human rights. This book is the beginning of this arduous work. I have shown that virtue, care, and feminist ethics form a cumulative argument in favor of ethical veganism. They have much to say about how we apply attention, care, and virtue to animals' experience of well-being and to recognizing that we are in a relationship with them, and the only consistent moral response is ethical veganism.

My argument began by criticizing the two major theories that started the discussion of how we should treat non-human animals. These two theories, utilitarianism and Kantian ethics, have proven inadequate at showing us that we should treat animals with respect. I discussed the limitations of Kantian and neo-Kantian ethics. These views are inadequate to frame a viable animal ethics. They propose that we have direct duty only toward rational beings; this exclude animals who, by their definition, are not rational. However, Kantians claim that we have indirect duties toward animals. This means that if I wrong an animal, my behavior causes other rational beings to promote the same attitude toward other rational beings. As I have argued, the problem with this formulation is that in order for a rational being to extrapolate wrong moral behavior toward animals and turn it toward rational beings, there must be something objective about the value of animals that might affect our behavior toward rational beings. But by their own definition, Kantians maintain that animals do not possess any objectively valuable characteristic. With regard to neo-Kantian theories, I argued that while they fix the problems in Kant's theory, they still are problematic. Essentially, people are not moved by the idea, nor are they convinced, that animals have rights or that we have obligations toward them. And even if such theories are correct—and people do not realize that they are wrong in not embracing those theories—there is nothing about such theories that can convince people to respect animals. As I have stated a number of times, such theories give reasons to act morally. On the other hand, the moral approach that I have proposed is that of a virtuous character, which is internally motivated.

Having shown that Kantianism is incapable of showing us that we should respect animals, I show that the alternative moral theory of utilitarianism is also inadequate for this purpose. Utilitarianism is the idea that the right action is one that, taking into consideration consequences, is capable of maximizing the overall utility. This approach is deficient because it demands too little of us. On the one hand it argues that we should respect animals because they have preferences; but on the other hand, utilitarianism discounts our moral feelings as genuine guides of morality. It tells us that our decision not to maltreat animals is to be determined by a utilitarian calculus that takes into consideration the satisfaction of preference for the greatest number of sentient beings. The problem with this approach to morality is that often in theorizing about what kind of consequences might satisfy the greatest number, we lose a great deal of important facts that we can only discover if we focus on the particular given situation and the lives and needs of particular individuals.

Having determined the inadequacy of utilitarianism and deontology to show us what is wrong with our treatment of animals, I propose a shift toward an ethic of virtue and care. These traditions emphasize the moral character of individuals rather than trying to determine the right moral action. Virtue ethics argues that this is a mistake. In fact, rules and principles come from external theories and give us prescriptions. But it is one thing to tell people what to do, and it is another thing to do something willingly and benevolently. A virtuous approach to morality says that we acquire important moral virtues through practice and we respond to particular situations by expressing these virtues.

With regard to our treatment of animals, many virtues are important, though I propose in particular compassion, fairness, temperance, and greatness of soul. These enable us to see what is morally virtuous about veganism. Ethical veganism is a worldview that wants us to realize that animals are not our property or our food; thus, we should not use them in any way. Compassion and fairness show that an individual endowed with these two virtues thoroughly understands the suffering of animals and tries to alleviate their suffering. Our behavior, specifically eating animals and using their by-products, causes unnecessary pain to animals. One cannot be, for example, a compassionate racist or a fair rapist. As compassion is rooted in love, one who is truly compassionate will act out of love, and there is nothing loving about racism. By the same token, one is not fair-minded if he is fair only to a restricted group of people or to his country, species, race, etc. To be fair means treating all equally. With regard to our treatment of non-human animals and our environment, a compassionate individual, by the very definition of compassion, desires to avoid that pain because he is interested in others' well-being. Veganism, then, is an expression of compassion. The compassionate individual refuses to take part in a practice centered on animal exploitation. And most importantly, one cannot be compassionate and use animals as means to one's ends. Compassionate killing, when it is done to eat an animal, is just an oxymoron. If I care for an animal and I am compassionate, by definition I make sure that that animal has a good life. Consequently it is absurd to believe that I care for a being but I intend to eat that being. If I care for a being, I will not do anything that could hurt her or use her body for food or clothing.

The virtue of temperance, as I have argued, is important especially in our society because the abundance of food and commodities is so high that people have lost sight of what is really necessary. Most people in the world eat for pleasure. This is not inherently wrong. However, the pleasure of food must harmonize with what is conducive to flourishing. As I have shown, when it comes to food, health sciences are very clear about nutrition: Animal-based food is counterproductive for human health while plant-based food is humans' optimal food—it improves our health, makes us thrive, and in many cases reverses chronic diseases. Thus, plant-based food is conducive to flourishing. A temperate individual, therefore, is one whose appetite is not regulated by the desire to satisfy cravings or taste; rather, the temperate individual chooses a diet devoid of animal products because they are not essential, they cause many health problems—thus hindering flourishing— and the taste is not such a vital factor that it cannot be overcome. Thus, temperance is conducive to ethical veganism.

The way I described ethical veganism—and thus the ethical vegan person—not surprisingly is the embodiment of virtue. I described the ethical vegan individual by using the name that Aristotle gave to the most important virtue: greatness of soul. The great-souled individual, a magnanimous person, is fair. The fair-minded behaves in a way that is consistently just. It is unfair to treat certain animals with respect and not others, and it is unfair to turn animals into food for the sake of taste, tradition, or just because we can, when those animals do not wish to become food. The magnanimous individual has the courage and sensibility to avoid all animal products because using animals, their body parts, and their secretions, is disgraceful. Using animals is not consistent with the actions of a great-souled person. Therefore, using animals as food, even when animals are treated "humanely," is wrong. Thus, virtue ethics can show us that the only morally good and consistent attitude toward our treatment of non-human animals and the environment is to embrace ethical veganism.

Bibliography

"6 Simple Ways to Be the Healthiest Vegan Ever." http://www.peta.org/living/food/vegetarian-101/vegans-guide-good-nutrition/.
Abbate, Cheryl. "Virtues and Animals: A Minimally Decent Ethic for Practical Living in Non-Ideal World." *Journal of Agricultural and Environmental Ethics* 27, no. 6 (2014).
Adams, Carol J. *The Sexual Politics of Meat: A Feminist-Vegetarian Critical Theory*. New York: Bloomsbury Academic, 2015.
———. "The Book." http://caroljadams.com/spom-the-book/.
Akhtar, Aysha. "The Flaws and Human Harms of Animal Experimentation." *Camb. Q. Healthc. Ethics* 24, no. 4 (October 2015): 407–419. doi:10.1017/S0963180115000079.
Aleksandrowicz, L., R. Green, E. J. M. Joy, P. Smith, A. Haines. "The Impacts of Dietary Change on Greenhouse Gas Emissions, Land Use, Water Use, and Health: A Systematic Review." *PLoS ONE* 11, no. 11 (2016): e0165797. https://doi.org/10.1371/journal.pone.0165797.
Allen, Colin. "Animal Pain." *Nous* 38, no. 4 (2004).
Allhoff, Francis. "What Is Modesty?" *International Journal of Applied Philosophy* 23, no. 2 (2010).
Alvaro, Carlo. "Ethical Veganism, Virtue, and Greatness of the Soul." *J. Agric. Environ. Ethics* 30 (2017): 765. https://doi.org/10.1007/s10806–017–9698-z.
———. "Veganism as a Virtue: How Compassion and Fairness Show Us What Is Virtuous about Veganism." *Future of Food: Journal of Food, Agriculture and Society* 5, no. 2 (2017).
Anderson, Elizabeth. "Animal Rights and the Values of Nonhuman Life." In *Animal Rights: Current Debates and New Directions*, ed. Cass R. Sunstein and Martha C. Nussbaum. Oxford: Oxford University Press, 2005.
Anderson, Eric C., and Lisa Feldman Barrett. "Affective Beliefs Influence the Experience of Eating Meat." *PLOS ONE*, August 24, 2016: e0160424. https://doi.org/10.1371/journal.pone.0160424, 2016.
"Animals Die Annually in Science Labs." http://www.heraldsun.com.au/news/victoria/more-than-600000-animals-die-annually-in-science-labs/news-story/aec0d7aa495fbd7b172b2fa933399b78, 2004.
Animals Used for Experimentation." http://www.peta.org/issues/animals-used-for-experimentation/.
Annas, Julia. *The Morality of Happiness*. Oxford: Oxford University Press, 1993.
Anscombe, G. E. M. "Modern Moral Philosophy." *Philosophy* 33, no. 124 (1958).
Aristotle. *Ars Rhetorica*, ed. W. D. Ross. Oxford: Clarendon Press, Oxford, 1959.
———. *De Arte Poetica*, ed. R. Kassel. Oxford: Clarendon Press, 1965.
———. *Nichomachean Ethics*. Cambridge: Cambridge University Press, 2000.

Arvan, Marcus. "Unifying the Categorical Imperative." *Southwest Philosophy Review* 28, no. 1 (2012).
Assessing the Environmental Impact of Consumption and Production." http://www.unep.org/resourcepanel/Portals/24102/PDFs/PriorityProductsAndMaterials_Report.pdf.
Ayer, J. Alfred. *Language, Truth and Logic*. New York: Dover Books, 1952.
BBC News. "Fraudster Bernard Madoff and Wife 'Attempted Suicide'" (2011). https://www.bbc.com/news/world-us-canada-15471683.
———. "World's First Lab-Grown Burger Is Eaten in London" (2013). https://www.bbc.com/news/science-environment-23576143.
Bentham, Jeremy. *An Introduction to the Principles of Morals and Legislation*. New York: Dover, 2007.
Ben-Ze'ev, Aaron. "The Virtue of Modesty." *American Philosophical Quarterly* 30 (1993).
Bernard, Neil. "1907 New York Times Article Shows that Meat Causes Cancer: A Century Later, Many People Still Haven't Heard the News" (2013). PCRM.org://www.pcrm.org/nbBlog/index.php/1907-new-york-times-article-shows-that-meat-causes-cancer-a-century-later-many.
———. *Dr. Neal Barnard's Program for Reversing Diabetes: The Scientifically Proven System for Reversing Diabetes without Drugs*. Emmaus, PA: Rodale Books, 2008.
Betti, Mirko, and Isah Datar. "Possibilities for an In Vitro Meat Production System." *Innovative Food Science and Emerging Technologies* 1 (2010): doi:10.1016/j.ifset.2009.10.007.
Bhat, Zuhaib Fayaz, Sunil Kumar, and Hina Fayaz. "In vitro meat production." *Journal of Integrative Agriculture* 14, no. 2 (February 2015): 246. https://doi.org/10.1016/S2095 3119(14)60887-X.
Bommarito, N. "Modesty as a Virtue of Attention." *Philosophical Review* 122, no. 1 (2013): 93–117. doi: 10.1215/00318108-1728723.
Bouvard, Véronique et al. "Carcinogenicity of Consumption of Red and Processed Meat" *The Lancet Oncology* 16, no. 16 (2015): 1599–1600.
Breindenbach, Bob. "Homeless Man Who Admitted to 23-Year-Old Unsolved Murder Gets 30 Years in Prison." *Providence Journal*. http://www.providencejournal.com/article/20150818/news/150819346.
Campbell, T. Colin. *The China Study: The Most Comprehensive Study of Nutrition Ever Conducted and the Startling Implications for Diet, Weight Loss, and Long-Term Health*. Dallas: BenBella Books, 2006.
Cancer Council NSW. "Meat and Cancer." https://www.cancercouncil.com.au/21639/cancer-prevention/diet-exercise/nutrition-diet/fruit-vegetables/meat-and-cancer/#ScVzbuPsBR pqsQZg.99, 2018.
"Cancer Increasing among Meat Eaters," *New York Times*, September 24, 1907. https://timesmachine.nytimes.com/timesmachine/1907/09/24/101857679.pdf. Retrieved on June 28, 2018.
Celona, Larry. "Bernie Madoff's Son, Mark, Commits Suicide." *The New York Post*, December 11, 2010. https://nypost.com/2010/12/11/bernie-madoffs-son-mark-commits-suicide.
Center for Biological Diversity. "How Eating Meat Hurts Wildlife and the Planet, Take Extinction off Your Plate." http://www.takeextinctionoffyourplate.com/meat_and_wildlife.html.
Chang-Claude, J., R. Frentzel-Beyme, and U. Eilber. "Mortality Patterns of German Vegetarians after 1 Years of Follow-Up." *Epidemiology* 3 (1992):395–401.
———. "Dietary and Lifestyle Determinants of Mortality among German Vegetarians." *Int. J. Epidemiol.* 22 (1993): 228–236.
Chappell, Tim. "In Defense of Speciesism." In *Human Lives: Critical Essays on Consequentialist Bioethics*, ed. David S. Odenberg and Jaqueline A. Laing. London: Macmillan, 1997.
Chatterjee, Deen. *The Ethics of Assistance*. Cambridge: Cambridge University Press, 2004.
Cohen, Carl. "The Case for the Use of Animals in Biomedical Research." *The New England Journal of Medicine* 315 (1986): 865–869.
Collins, Nick. "Test Tube Hamburgers to Be Served This Year," *The Telegraph*, February 19, 2012. https://www.telegraph.co.uk/news/science/science-news/9091628/Test-tube-hamburgers-to-be-served-this-year.html.

Coogan, Michael D., ed. *New Oxford Annotated Bible: New Revised Standard Version with the Apocryphal/Deuterocanonical Books*. New York: Oxford University Press, 2001.
Cornell Chronicle. "U.S. Could Feed 800 Million People with Grain That Livestock Eat, Cornell Ecologist Advises Animal Scientists," August 7, 1997. http://news.cornell.edu/stories/1997/08/us-could-feed-800-million-people-grain-livestock-eat.
Cory, Lloyd. *Quote Unquote*. Victor Books, 1977.
Cox, Christopher. "Consider the Oyster: Why Even Strict Vegans Should Feel Comfortable Eating Oysters by the Boatload." *Slate*, April 7, 2010. http://www.slate.com/articles/life/food/2010/04/consider_the_oyster.html. Retrieved on June 27, 2018.
Craig, W. J., and A. R. Mangels. "Position of the American Dietetic Association: Vegetarian Diets." *Am. Diet. Assoc.* 109, no. 7 (2009): 1266–82.
Crary, Alice. *Inside Ethics: On the Demands of Moral Thought*. Cambridge, MA: Harvard University Press, 2016.
Crisp, Roger. "Aristotle on Greatness of Soul." In *The Blackwell Guide to Aristotle's Nicomachean Ethics*, ed. R. Kraut. Oxford: Blackwell Publishing, 2006.
———. "Compassion and Beyond." *Ethical Theory and Moral Practice* 11, no. 3 (2008). Papers Presented at the Annual Conference of the British Society for Ethical Theory, Bristol.
"Current Eating Patterns in the United States." *Dietary Guidelines 2015-2020* (2015). https://health.gov/dietaryguidelines/2015/guidelines/chapter-2/current-eating-patterns-in-the-united-states/#current-eating-patterns-in-the-united-states.
de Boo, Jasmijn. "The Future of Food, Why Lab Grown Meat Is Not the Solution." *Huffpost*, September 8, 2013. https://www.huffingtonpost.co.uk/jasmijn-de-boo/lab-grown-meat_b_3730367.html.
DeGrazia, David. *Taking Animals Seriously: Mental Life and Moral Status*. Cambridge: Cambridge University Press, 1996.
de Lazari-Radek, Katarzyna, and Peter Singer. *The Point of View of the Universe: Sidgwick and Contemporary Ethics*. Oxford: Oxford University Press, 2014.
Denis, Lara. "Kant's Conception of Duties regarding Animals: Reconstruction and Reconsideration." *History of Philosophy Quarterly* 17, no. 4 (October 2000).
Descartes, René. *Discourse on Method, Optics, Geometry, and Meteorology*, trans. Paul J. Olscamp. Indianapolis: Bobbs-Merrill, 1965.
———. "Letter to Marquess of Newcastle, 23 November, 1646." In *Descartes' Philosophical Letters*, translated and edited by Anthony Kenny. Oxford: Clarendon Press, 1970.
d'Holbach, Baron Paul. "Of the System of Man's Free Agency." In *System of Nature*, 1770.
Diamond, Cora. "Eating Meat and Eating People." *Philosophy* 53, no. 206 (1978).
Donovan, Josephine. "Feminism and the Treatment of Animals: From Care to Dialogue."*Signs* 31, no. 2 (2006).
Donovan, Josephine, and Carol J. Adams. *The Feminist Care Tradition in Animal Ethics*. New York: Columbia University Press, 2007.
Driver, Julia. "The Virtues of Ignorance." *The Journal of Philosophy* 86, no. 7 (1989): 373–84. doi:10.230/20027146.
———. *Uneasy Virtue*. New York: Cambridge University Press, 2001.
Drouin, G., J. R. Godin, and B. Pagé. "The Genetics of Vitamin C Loss in Vertebrates." doi:10.2174/138920211796429736.
Duhaime-Ross, Arielle. "Test-Tube Burger: Lab-Cultured Meat Passes Taste Test (Sort of)." *Scientific American*, August 5, 2013. https://www.scientificamerican.com/article/test-tube-burger-lab-culture/.
"Egg Industry Grinds Millions of Baby Chicks Alive." https://www.youtube.com/watch?v=BQ5qAfyUuWE by HoTvid. Retrieved on June 19, 2018.
The_Einsteinian_God, "Would Meat Grown in a Lab Change Your Mind about Eating Meat?" *Reddit*, accessed August 23, 2018. https://www.reddit.com/user/the_einsteinian_god.
Engster, Daniel. "Care Ethics and Animal Welfare." *Journal of Social Philosophy* 37, no. 4 (2006).
Environmental Protection Agency. "What's the Problem? Animal Waste Region 9 US EPA." https://www.epa.gov/.

Environmental Working Group. "Meat Eater's Guide." https://www.ewg.org/meateatersguide/interactive-graphic/meat-consumption/.

———. "Water." https://www.ewg.org/meateatersguide/interactive-graphic/water/.

Fessler, Daniel M. T. et al. "Disgust Sensitivity and Meat Consumption: A Test of an Emotivist Account of Moral Vegetarianism." *Appetite* 41, no. 1 (2003): 31–41.

"The Flaws and Human Harms of Animal Experimentation." *Camb. Q. Healthc. Ethics.* 24, no. 4 (October 2015): 407–419. doi:10.1017/S0963180115000079.

Fleischman, Diana. "Lab Meat: Survey Results," *The Vegan Option Radio Show and Blog* (May 16, 2012). Accessed June 12, 2018. https://theveganoption.org/2012/05/16/lab-meat-survey-results/.

Foot, Philippa. *Natural Goodness.* Oxford: Clarendon Press, 2001.

———. "Virtue and Vices." In *Virtues and Vices and Other Essays in Moral Philosophy*, 1–18. Oxford: Clarendon Press, 1979.

Fraser, G., and E. Haddad. "Hot Topic: Vegetarianism, Mortality and Metabolic Risk: The New Adventist Health Study." Report presented at Academy of Nutrition and Dietetic (Food and Nutrition Conference) Annual Meeting, October 7, 2012, Philadelphia, PA.

Frede, Dorothea. "The Historic Decline of Virtue Ethics." In *The Cambridge Companion to Virtue Ethics.* Cambridge: Cambridge University Press, 2013.

Frey, G. R. "The Case against Animal Rights." In *Animal Rights and Human Obligations*, ed. Tom Regan and Peter Singer. Upper Saddle River, NJ: Prentice-Hall, 1989.

Gajdusek, D. C., and V. Zigas. "Degenerative Disease of the Central Nervous System in New Guinea: The Endemic Occurrence of "Kuru" in the Native Population." *New Engl. J. Med.* 257 (1957): 974–978.

Geach, Peter. *The Virtues: The Stanton Lectures 1973–74.* Cambridge: Cambridge University Press, 1977.

Gerbens-Leenes, P. W., M. M. Mekonnen, and A. Y. Hoekstra. "The Water Footprint of Poultry, Pork and Beef: A Comparative Study in Different Countries and Production Systems." *Water Resources and Industry, Water Footprint Assessment (WFA) for Better Water Governance and Sustainable Development* 1–2 (March 2013): 25–36. doi:10.1016/j.wri.2013.03.001.

Gibson, Boyce. *The Philosophy of Descartes.* London: Methuen, 1932.

Goodland, Robert, and Jeff Anhang. "Livestock and Climate Change." Worldwatch Institute. (2018). http://www.worldwatch.org/node/6294.

Gordon, I. *Reproductive Technologies in Farm Animals.* CABI. 2004.

Griffin, Donald R. *Animal Minds Beyond Cognition to Consciousness,* Chicago: University of Chicago Press, 2001.

Gruen, Lori. "Empathy and Vegetarian Commitments." *The Feminist Tradition in Animal Ethics.* New York: Columbia University Press, 2007.

———. *Entangled Empathy: An Alternative Ethic for Our Relationship with Animals.* New York: Lantern Books, 2014.

Halwani, Raja. "Care Ethics and Virtue Ethics." *Hypatia* 18, no. 3 (2003): 161–192.

Hare, Richard M. *Moral Thinking: Its Levels, Method, and Point.* Oxford: Oxford University Press, 1982.

Harvard Health Publishing. "Halt Heart Disease with a Plant-Based, Oil-Free Diet." (September 2014). https://www.health.harvard.edu/heart-health/halt-heart-disease-with-a-plant-based-oil-free-diet-.

Harvard T. H. Chan School of Public Health. "Red Meat Consumption and Breast Cancer Risk." (2018). https://www.hsph.harvard.edu/news/features/red-meat-consumption-and-breast-cancer-risk/.

———. "Vegetables and Fruit." https://www.hsph.harvard.edu/nutritionsource/what-should-you-eat/vegetables-and-fruits/.

Hawks, Charlotte. "How Close Are We to a Hamburger Grown in a Lab?" CNN. https://www.cnn.com/2018/03/01/health/clean-in-vitro-meat-food/index.html.

Held, Virginia. *The Ethics of Care: Personal, Political, and Global.* Oxford: Oxford University Press 2007.

Herman, Barbara. *The Practice of Moral Judgement*. Cambridge: Harvard University Press, 1993.

Herrero, Mario, et al. "Biomass Use, Production, Feed Efficiencies, and Greenhouse Gas Emissions from Global Livestock Systems." Proceedings of the National Academy of Sciences 110, no. 52 (December 24, 2013): 20888–93. doi:10.1073/pnas.1308149110.

Hocquette, J. F. "Is In Vitro Meat the Solution for the Future?" *Meat Sci.* 120 (October 2016): 167–176. doi: 10.1016/j.meatsci.2016.04.036.

The Holy Bible: Containing the Old and New Testaments—New King James Version. Nelson Bibles, 2005.

The Human Society. "Question and Answers about Biomedical Research." http://www.humanesociety.org/issues/biomedical_research/qa/questions_answers.html. Retrieved on June 18, 2018.

Hursthouse, Rosalind. "Applying Virtue Ethics to Our Treatment of Other Animals." In *The Practice of Virtue: Classic and Contemporary Readings in Virtue Ethics*, ed. J. Welchman Jennifer. Indianapolis, IN: Hackett Publishing, 2006.

———. "Normative Virtue Ethics." In *How Should One Live?*, ed. Roger Crisp. Oxford: Oxford University Press, 1996.

———. "Virtue Ethics and the Treatment of Animals." In *The Oxford Handbook of Animal Ethics*, ed. T. Beauchamp and R. Frey Oxford: Oxford University Press, 2011.

———. "Virtue Theory and Abortion," *Philosophy & Public Affairs* 20, no. 3 (1991).

———. *On Virtue Ethics*. Oxford: Oxford University Press, 1999.

Hussar, K. M., and P. L. Harris. "Children Who Choose Not to Eat Meat: A Study of Early Moral Decision-Making." *Social Development* 19 (2010): 627–641. doi:10.1111/j.1467-9507.2009.00547.x.

Institute of Agriculture and Natural Resources. "How Much Water Do Cows Drink per Day?" (2016).

———. "The Water Content of Things: How Much Water Does It Take to Grow a Hamburger?" (2016). https://water.usgs.gov/edu/activity-watercontent.php.

Inuit Cultural Online Resource. "Modern vs. Traditional Life: Explore our Culture, Modern vs. Traditional Life." https://www.icor.ottawainuitchildrens.com/explore-our-culture. Retrieved on June 27, 2018.

Institute of Medicine and National Research Council. *U.S. Health in International Perspective: Shorter Lives, Poorer Health*. Washington, DC: National Academies Press, 2013.

"Is It OK to Eat Eggs from Chickens I've Raised in My Backyard?" http://www.peta.org/about-peta/faq/is-it-ok-to-eat-eggs-from-chickens-ive-raised-in-my-backyard/.

Jha, Alok. "Synthetic Meat: How the World's Costliest Burger Made It on to the Plate." *The Guardian*, August 5, 2013. https://www.theguardian.com/science/2013/aug/05/synthetic-meat-burger-stem-cells.

Jochems, Carlo, et al., "The Use of Fetal Bovine Serum: Ethical or Scientific Problem?," ATLA-Nottingham 30, no. 2 (2002).

Johns Hopkins Bloomberg School of Public Health. "Health & Environmental Implications of U.S. Meat Consumption & Production." https://www.jhsph.edu/research/centers-and-institutes/johns-hopkins-center-for-a-livable-future/projects/meatless_monday/resources/meat_consumption.html.

Johnson, Edward. "Life, Death, and Animals" In *Ethics and Animals: Contemporary Issues in Biomedicine, Ethics, and Society*, ed. H. B. Miller and W. H. Williams W.H. New York: Humana Press, 1983.

Jouvet, D., P. Vimont, F. Delorme, and M. Jouvet. "Study of Selective Deprivation of the Paradoxal Sleep Phase in the Cat." *C. R. Seances Soc. Biol. Fil.* (in French) (1964).

Joy, Melanie. "Dis-ease of the Heart: The Psychology of Eating Animals." *Forks over Knives*, May 23, 2012. https://www.forksoverknives.com/dis-ease-of-the-heart-the-psychology-of-eating-animals/#gs.=G3q7lw.

———. *Why We Love Dogs, Eat Pigs, and Wear Cows: An Introduction to Carnism*. Newburyprot, MA: Conari Press, 2011.

———. "What Is Carnism?" https://www.carnism.org/carnism.

Kant, Immanuel. *The Groundwork for the Metaphysics of Morals* (1785), trans. Mary J. Gregor. Cambridge: Cambridge University Press, 2013.

———. *Lectures on Ethics*, trans. Louis Infield. New York: Harper and Row, 1963.

———. *Lectures on Anthropology: The Cambridge Edition of the Works of Immanuel Kant*, translated by Robert B. Louden. Cambridge: Cambridge University Press, 2013.

———. *The Metaphysics of Morals*. In *Practical Philosophy*, ed. and trans. M. J. Gregor. Cambridge: Cambridge University Press, 1996.

———. "Religion within the Limits of Reason Alone." In *Religion and Rational Theology*. Cambridge: Cambridge University Press, 2001.

Kass, Leon R. "The Wisdom of Repugnance." *The New Republic* 216, no. 22 (1997): 20.

Khan, K. S. "Comparison of Treatment Effects between Animal Experiments and Clinical Trials: Systematic Review." *BMJ* (2007).

"Kings of the Carnivores: Who Eats Most Meat?" *The Economist* (April 30, 2012). https://www.economist.com/graphic-detail/2012/04/30/kings-of-the-carnivores.

Kittay, Eva Feder, and Licia Carlson, eds. *Cognitive Disability and Its Challenge to Moral Philosophy*. Hoboken, NJ: Wiley-Blackwell, 2010.

Korsgaard, Christine. "Fellow Creatures: Kantian Ethics and Our Duties to Animals." *The Sources of Normativity*. Cambridge: Cambridge University Press, 2005.

———. "Kant's Formula of Universal Law." *Pacific Philosophical Quarterly* 66, no. 1–2 (1985).

Kuhse, H., and P. Singer. "Doctors' Practices and Attitudes Regarding Voluntary Euthanasia." *Med. J. Aust* (1988).

Kupperman, J. Joel. "A Messy Derivation of the Categorical Imperative." *Philosophy* 77 (2002).

Louden, Robert. "Some Vices of Virtue Ethics." In *Ethical Theory Classic and Contemporary Readings*, ed. Louis Pojman (1989).

Louisiana Universities Marine Consortium. "Press Release," August 4, 2014. https://www2.fgcu.edu/swamp/files/Hypoxia_Press_Release_2014.pdf.

Luke, Brian. "Justice, Caring and Animal Liberation." In *The Feminist Care Tradition in Animal Ethics*, 124–148. Columbia: Columbia University Press, 2007.

Mackie, J. Leslie. *Ethics: Inventing Right and Wrong*. New York: Penguin, 1977.

Maes, Hans. "Modesty, Asymmetry, and Hypocrisy." *Journal of Value Inquiry* 38, no. 4 (2004): 485–97. doi: 10.1007/s10790–005–3335–1.

Malisow, Craig. "Tens of Thousands of Dogs Are Still Used in Laboratory Testing Every Year." *Houston Press*, May 4, 2015. http://www.houstonpress.com/news/tens-of-thousands-of-dogs-are-still-used-in-laboratory-testing-every-year-7400834.Retrieved on June 23, 2018.

Margulis, Sérgio. "Causes of Deforestation of the Brazilian Amazon." World Bank Working Paper, no. 22 (2004).

Matheny, Gaverick. "Expected Utility, Contributory Causation, and Vegetarianism." *Journal of Applied Philosophy* 19 (2002).

———. "Utilitarianism and Animals." In *In Defense of Animals: The Second Wave*, ed. P. Singer. Malden: Blackwell, 2002.

Matthews, R. A. "Medical Progress Depends on Animal Models—Doesn't It?" *J. R. Soc. Med.* (2008).

Mattick, Carolyn, et al. "Anticipatory Life Cycle Analysis of In Vitro Biomass Cultivation for Cultured Meat Production in the United States." *Environmental Science & Technology* 49, no. 19 (October 6, 2015): 11941–49. doi:10.1021/acs.est.5b01614.

———. "The Problem with Making Meat in a Factory." *Slate*, September 28, 2015. http://www.slate.com/articles/technology/future_tense/2015/09/in_vitro_meat_probably_won_t_save_the_planet_yet.html.

Mattick, Carolyn, and Brad Allenby. "The Future of Meat: Issues in Science and Technology." *Issues in Science and Technology* 30, no. 1 (2013).

Maulvault, Ana Luísa, Patrícia Anacleto, Vera Barbosa, et al. "Toxic Elements and Speciation in Seafood Samples from Different Contaminated Sites in Europe." *Environmental Research* 143, part B (November 2015). https://doi.org/10.1016/j.envres.2015.09.016.

McDougall, Christopher. *Born to Run: A Hidden Tribe, Superathletes, and the Greatest Race the World Has Never Seen*. New York: Vintage, 2011.
McDowell, John. "Two Sorts of Naturalism." In *Virtues and Reasons: Philippa Foot and Moral Theory: Essays in Honour of Philippa Foot*, ed. Rosalind Hursthouse, Gavin Lawrence, and Warren Quinn. Oxford: Oxford University Press, 1998.
McLaren, Margaret. "Feminist Ethics: Care as a Virtue." In *Feminists Doing Ethics*. Lanham, MD: Rowman and Littlefield, 2001.
McMullin, Irene. "A Modest Proposal: Accounting for the Virtuousness of Modesty." *The Philosophical Quarterly* 60 (2010).
McPherson, Tristram. "A Case for Ethical Veganism." *Journal of Moral Philosophy* 11, no. 6 (2014): 677–703.
———. "Why I Am a Vegan (and You Should Be One Too)." In *Philosophy Comes to Dinner*. Abingdon, UK: Routledge, 2015.
Mesfin, M. Mekonnen, and Arjen Y. Hoekstra. "A Global Assessment of the Water Footprint of Farm Animal Products." *Ecosystems* 15, no. 3 (2012). doi:10.1007/s10021–011–9517–8.
Midgley, Mary. *Animals and Why They Matter*. Athens, GA: The University of Georgia Press, 1983.
———. "Biotechnology and Monstrosity: Why We Should Pay Attention to the 'Yuk Factor'" *Hastings Center Report* 30, no. 5 (2000).
Mill, John Stuart. *Utilitarianism* (1863). London: Parker, Son & Bourn, 2002.
Montalcini, T., D. De Bonis, Y. Ferro, et al. "High Vegetable Fats Intake Is Associated With High Resting Energy Expenditure in Vegetarians." *Nutrients* 7, no. 7 (2015). https://doi.org/10.3390/nu7075259.
Murdoch, Iris. "The Idea of Perfection." In *The Sovereignty of The Good*. London: Routledge, 1970.
Murphy, Marc. "Book Review." *Ethics* 113, no. 2 (2003).
NBCPhiladelphia.com. "Man Who Confessed to 1990 Murder Gets 30 Years." July 19, 2013. https://www.nbcphiladelphia.com/news/local/Man-Who-Confessed-to-23-Year-Old-Murder-Gets-30-Years-216182991.html. Retreived on June 15, 2018.
Noddings, Nel. *Caring: A Feminine Approach to Ethics and Moral Education*. Berkeley: University of California Press, 1984.
Nolt, John. "The Move from Good to Ought." *Environmental Ethics* 28, no. 4, 2006.
Nussbaum, M. "Danger to Human Dignity." *The Chronicle of Higher Education* (2004). https://www.chronicle.com/article/Danger-to-Human-Dignity-the/21047.
"Obesity Information." http://www.heart.org/ HEARTORG/Healthy Living/WeightManagement/Obesity/Obesity-Information_UCM_307908_Article.jsp#.WGci9bGZNE4.
O'Neill, Onora. "Consistency in action." *Constructions of Reason: Exploration of Kant's Political Philosophy*. Cambridge/New York: Cambridge University Press, 1989.
Oppenlander, Richard. *Food Choice and Sustainability: Why Buying Local, Eating Less Meat, and Taking Baby Steps Won't Work*. Minneapolis: Langdon Street Press, 2013.
———. "Freshwater Abuse and Loss: Where Is It All Going?" *Forks over Knives*, May 20, 2013. https://www.forksoverknives.com/freshwater-abuse-and-loss-where-is-it-all-going/#gs.MssSirQ.
Orlich, M. J., P. N. Singh, J. Sabaté, et al. "Vegetarian Dietary Patterns and Mortality in Adventist Health Study 2." *JAMA Intern. Med.* 173, no. 13 (2013): 1230–1238. doi:10.1001/jamainternmed.2013.6473.
Pachirat, Timothy. *Every Twelve Seconds: Industrialized Slaughter and the Politics of Sight*. New Haven, CT: Yale University Press, 2013.
PCRM. "Meat Consumption and Cancer Risk." http://www.pcrm.org/health/cancer-resources/diet-cancer/facts/meat-consumption-and-cancer-risk.
Pelegrines, N. *Theodosios Kant's Conceptions of the Categorical Imperative and the Will*. London: Zeno, 1980.
Pence, E. Gregory. *Classic Cases in Medical Ethics: Accounts of Cases That Have Shaped Medical Ethics, with Philosophical, Legal, and Historical Backgrounds*. New York: McGraw-Hill Humanities/Social Sciences/Languages, 2003.
———. *Medical Ethics*. New York: McGraw-Hill Education, 2014.

Perel, P., I. Roberts, E. Sena, P. Wheble, et al. "Comparison of Treatment Effects between Animal Experiments and Clinical Trials: Systematic Review." *BMJ* (2007).

PETA. "Animals Used for Experimentation." https://www.peta.org/issues/animals-used-for-experimentation/.

———. "Is It OK to Eat Eggs from Chickens I've Raised in My Backyard?" http://www.peta.org/about-peta/faq/is-it-ok-to-eat-eggs-from-chickens-ive-raised-in-my-backyard/.

Phillips, R. L. "Role of Lifestyle and Dietary Habits in Risk of Cancer among Seventh-Day Adventists." *Cancer Res.* 35 (1975): 3513–3522.

Phillips, Ashley. "PETA Offers $1M Prize for Lab-Grown Meat." ABCNews, April 23, 2008, https://abcnews.go.com/Technology/story?id=4704447&page=1.

Plato. *Euthyphro* and *Crito*. In *Five Dialogues: Euthyphro, Apology, Crito, Meno, Phaedo*, ed. John M. Cooper, trans. G. M. A. Grube. Indiannapolis: Hackett Publishing Company, 2002.

———. *Republic*, trans. C. D. C. Reeve. Indiannapolis: Hackett Publishing Company, 2004.

Pojman, Louis, and Lewis Vaughn. *Philosophy: The Quest for Truth*.

Preece, Gordon, "The Unthinkable & Unbelievable Singer" in *Rethinking Peter Singer: A Christian Critique*, Gordon Preece, ed. Downers Grove, Ill. InterVarsity Press, 2002.

———., ed. *Rethinking Peter Singer: A Christian Critique*. Downers Grove, IL: InterVarsity Press, 2002.

Premack, Rachel. "Meat is Horrible." *The Washington Post*, July 3, 2016. https://www.washingtonpost.com/news/wonk/wp/2016/06/30/how-meat-is-destroying-the-planet-in-seven-charts/?utm_term=.fa399b2b7544.

Pribis, P., R. C. Pencak, and T. Grajales. "Beliefs and Attitudes toward Vegetarian Lifestyle across Generations." *Nutrients* 2, no. 5 (2010).

Putman, Daniel "Relational Ethics and Virtue Ethics." *Metaphilosophy* 22 (1991).

"Questions and Answers about Biomedical Research." http://www.humanesociety.org/issues/biomedical_research/qa/questions_answers.html.

Quora. "When Do Kids Realize That Eating Meat Involves Killing Animals?" https://www.quora.com/When-do-kids-realize-that-eating-meat-involves-killing-animals. Retrieved on June 27, 2018.

Qur'an. Oxford: Oxford University Press, 2008.

Rachels, James. "The Challenge of Cultural Relativism." In *Ethics: Essential Readings in Moral Theory*. London: Routledge, 2012.

———. *Created from Animals: The Moral Implications of Darwinism*. Oxford: Oxford University Press, 1991.

Rachels, James, and Stuart Rachels. *Problems from Philosophy*, 2nd ed. New York: McGraw-Hill, 2005.

Regan, Tom. *The Case for Animal Rights*. Berkeley, CA: University of California Press, 1983.

———. "The Case for Animal Rights." In *In Defense of Animals*, ed. Peter Singer. New York: Basil Blackwell, 1985.

———. *The Thee Generation: Reflections of the Coming Revolution*. Philadelphia: Temple University Press, 1991.

Regan, Tom, and Peter Singer, eds. *Animal Rights and Human Obligations*. Englewood Cliffs: Prentice-Hall, 1989.

Research Council (US); Institute of Medicine (US); Woolf SH, Aron L, editors. Washington (DC): National Academies Press (US), 2013.

Roberts, W. C. "Twenty Questions on Atherosclerosis." *Proceedings* (Baylor University Medical Center) 13, no. 2 (2000): 139–143.

Roeder, Amy. "Red Meat Consumption and Breast Cancer Risk," October 9, 2014, https://www.hsph.harvard.edu/news/features/red-meat-consumption-and-breast-cancer-risk/

Russell, C. Daniel. *The Cambridge Companion to Virtue Ethics*. Cambridge: Cambridge University Press, 2013.

———. "Virtue Ethics in Modern Moral Philosophy." In *The Cambridge Companion to Virtue Ethics*. Cambridge: Cambridge University Press, 2013.

Saunders, J. Debra. "One Man's Animal Husbandry." *SFGATE*, March 20, 2001. Retreived on June 28, 2018. https://www.sfgate.com/opinion/saunders/article/One-Man-s-Animal-Husbandry-3316192.php.

Schaefer, G. O., and J. Savulescu. "The Ethics of Producing In Vitro Meat." *Journal of Applied Philosophy*, 31, no. 2 (2014): 188–202. http://doi.org/10.1111/japp.12056.

Schaubroeck, Katrien. "Interview with Christine Korsgaard, Holder of the Cardinal Mercier Chair 2009," *The Leuven Philosophy Newsletter* 17 (2008-2009/2009-2010).

Scheer, Roddy, and Doug Moss. "How Does Meat in the Diet Take an Environmental Toll?" *Scientific American*. https://www.scientificamerican.com/article/meat-and-environment/.

Schueler, G. F. "Why Modesty Is a Virtue." *Ethics* 107, no. 3 (1997).

Schweitzer, Albert. *Civilization and Ethics* (Part II of *The Philosophy of Civilization*) In *Animal Rights and Human Obligations*, ed. Tom Regan and Peter Singer. Upper Saddle River, NJ: Prentice Hall, 1989.

———. "The Ethic of Reverence for Life," in *Animal Rights and Human Obligations*, ed. Tom Regan and Peter Singer. Englewood Cliffs: Prentice Hall, 1989.

Seligman, E. P. Martin. "Learned Helplessness." *Annual Review of Medicine* 23 (1972): 407–412.

Seventh-Day Adventist Church. "Living a Healthful Life." https://www.adventist.org/en/vitality/health/. Retreived on June 27, 2018.

Shafer-Landau, Russell. "Vegetarianism, Causation and Ethical Theory." *Public Affairs Quarterly* 8, no. 1 (1994).

Singer, Peter. "All Animals Are Equal." *Philosophic Exchange* 5, no. 1 (1974).

———. *Animal Liberation: A New Ethics for Our Treatment of Animals*. New York: Random House, 1975.

———. *The Expanding Circle: Ethics and Sociology*. New York: Farrar, Straus, and Giroux, 1981.

———, ed. *In Defense of Animals*. New York: Basil Blackwell, 1985.

———. "What Causes Ocean 'Dead Zones'?" *Scientific American*. https://www.scientificamerican.com/article/ocean-dead-zones/. Retreived on June 29, 2018.

———. *Practical Ethics*, 2nd ed. Cambridge: Cambridge University Press, 1993.

———. "Utilitarianism and Vegetarianism." *Philosophy and Public Affairs* 9, no. 4 (1980): 305–324.

Singer, Peter, and Katarzyna de Lazari-Radek. *The Point of View of the Universe*. Oxford: Oxford University Press, 2016.

Singer, Peter, and Helsa Kuhse. "More On Euthanasia: A Response To Pauer-Studer," *The Monist* 76, no. 2 (1993): 158-174.

Slavin, J. L., and B. Lloyd. "Health Benefits of Fruits and Vegetables." *Advances in Nutrition* 3, no. 4 (2012): 506–516. http://doi.org/10.3945/an.112.002154.

Slicer, Deborah. "Your Daughter or Your Dog? A Feminist Assessment of the Animal Research Issue." In *The Feminist Care Tradition in Animal Ethics: A Reader*, ed. Josephine Donovan and Carol J. Adams. New York: Columbia University Press, 2007.

Sinsheimer, Robert L. "The Prospect of Designed Genetic Change." *Engineering and Science* 32, no. 7 (1969): 8–13. ISSN 0013–7812.

Slote, Michael. *The Impossibility of Perfection: Aristotle, Feminism, and the Complexities of Ethics*. New York: Oxford University Press, 2011.

———. *Morals from Motives*. Oxford: Oxford University Press, 2001.

———. *Moral Sentimentalism*. New York: Oxford University Press, 2010.

———. "Virtue Ethics." In *Three Methods of Ethics*, ed. Marcia Baron, Philip Pettit, and Michael Slote, 175–238. Oxford: Blackwell, 1997.

———. "Virtue Ethics and Democratic Values." *Journal of Social Philosophy* 14 (1993): 5–37.

Smith, A. Jane. "A Question of Pain in Invertebrates," *ILAR Journal* 33, no. 1–2 (1991).

Smith, N. Kemp. *New Studies in the Philosophy of Descartes*. London: Macmillan, 1952.

Smith, P., M. Bustamante, H. Ahammad, H. Clark, H. Dong, E. A. Elsiddig, H. Haberl, R. Harper, J. House, M. Jafari, O. Masera, C. Mbow, N. H. Ravindranath, C. W. Rice, C. R. Abad, A. Romanovskaya, F. Sperling, F. N. Tubiello, S. Bolwig. "Agriculture, Forestry and

Other Land Use (AFOLU)." In *Climate Change 2014: Mitigation of Climate Change*. Cambridge: Cambridge University Press, 2014.

Snowdon, Kathryn. "Why Every Day Needs to Be World Animal Day," October 4, 2016. http://aavs.org/animals-science/how-animals-are-used/testing/.

Specter, M. "Test-Tube Burgers." *The New Yorker* https://www.newyorker.com/magazine/2011/05/23/test-tube-burgers.

Specter, Michael. "The Dangerous Philosopher." *The New Yorker*, September 6, 1999.

St. Augustine. *The Confessions*. New York: Vintage, 1998.

Statman, Daniel. "Modesty, Pride and Realistic Self-Assessment." *The Philosophical Quarterly* 42, no. 169 (1992): 420–38. doi: 10.2307/2220284.

Steinfeld, Henning, Pierre Gerber, Tom Wassenaar, Vincent Castel, and Mauricio Rosales. "Livestock's Long Shadow." *Food And Agriculture Organization Of The United Nations*. http://www.europarl.europa.eu/climatechange/doc/FAO%20report%20executive%20summary.pdf.

Stephens, O. William. "Five Arguments for Vegetarianism." *Philosophy in the Contemporary World* 1, no. 4 (1994): 25–39.

Stocker, Michael. "The Schizophrenia of Modern Moral Theories." *Journal of Philosophy* 73 (1976).

Swanton, Christine. "The Definition of Virtue Ethics." In *The Cambridge Companion to Virtue Ethics*, 315–338. Cambridge: Cambridge University Press, 2003.

Taylor, Richard. *Good and Evil*. Amherst, NY: Prometheus Books, 1999.

"Tens of Thousands of Dogs Are Still Used in Laboratory Testing Every Year." http://www.houstonpress.com/news/tens-of-thousands-of-dogs-are-still-used-in-laboratory-testing-every-year-7400834.

Tharrey, Marion, et. al. "Patterns of Plant and Animal Protein Intake Are Strongly Associated with Cardiovascular Mortality: The Adventist Health Study-2 Cohort." https://doi.org/10.1093/ije/dyy030.

Thomas, Alan. "Virtue Ethics and an Ethics of Care: Complementary or in Conflict?" *Eidos: Revista de Filosofía de la Universidad del Norte* 14 (2011).

Thornton, Philip, Mario Herrero, and Polly Ericksen. "Livestock and Climate Change." International Livestock Research Institute (2011). [cgspace.Cgiar.org/bitstream/handle/10568/10601/IssueBrief3. Pdf].

Thorogood, M., J. Mann, P. Appleby, and K. McPherson. "Risk of Death from Cancer and Ischaemic Heart Disease in Meat and Non-Meat Eaters." *Br. Med. J.* 308 (1994): 1667–1670.

ThoughtCo. "What is Veganism? What Do Vegans Eat, and from What Do They Abstain?" https://www.thoughtco.com/what-is-veganism-127598. Retreived on June 26, 2018.

Tooley, Michael. "Abortion and Infanticide." *Philosophy and Public Affairs* 2, no. 1 (1972): 37–65.

"Trends in Meat Consumption in the United States." *Public Health Nutr.* 14, no. 4 (2011): 575–583. doi: 10.1017/S1368980010002077.

Tuomisto, Hanna L., and M. Joost Teixeira de Mattos. "Environmental Impacts of Cultured Meat Production." *Environmental Science & Technology* 45, no. 14 (July 15, 2011): 6117–23. doi:10.1021/es200130u.

Tuso, P. J., M. H. Ismail, B. P. Ha, C. Bartolotto. "Nutritional Update for Physicians: Plant-Based Diets." *The Permanente Journal* 17, no. 2 (2013): 61–66. doi:10.7812/TPP/12–085.

Two and a Half Men, "My Tongue Is Meat." CBS, February 27, 2006, episode 15, season 3.

UN Convention to Combat Desertification, "New ISO Standard to Combat Land Degradation." June 11, 2017. https://knowledge.unccd.int/publications/new-iso-standard-combat-land-degradation. Retreived on June 27, 2018.

UNEP. "Assessing the Environmental Impacts of Consumption and Production: Priority Products and Materials." A Report of the Working Group on the Environmental Impacts of Products and Materials to the International Panel for Sustainable Resource Management. Hertwich, E., van der Voet, E., Suh, S., Tukker, A., Huijbregts M., Kazmicrczyk, P., Lenzen, M., McNeely, J., Moriguchi, Y.

UNICEF. "Improving Child Nutrition." https://www.unicef.org/gambia/Improving_Child_Nutrition_the_achievable_imperative_for_global_progress.pdf.
University of Southern California. "Meat and Cheese May Be as Bad for You as Smoking." *ScienceDaily*. www.sciencedaily.com/releases/2014/03/140304125639.htm. Accessed June 20, 2018.
The U.S. Environmental Protection Agency. *National Enforcement Initiative: Preventing Animal Waste from Contaminating Surface and Ground Water*. https://www.epa.gov/enforcement/national-enforcement-initiative-preventing-animal-waste-contaminating-surface-and-ground.
The USGS Water Science School. "The Water Content of Things: How Much Water Does It Take to Grow a Hamburger?" https://water.usgs.gov/edu/activity-watercontent.php. Retrieved on June 21, 2018.
U.S. Department of Agriculture, Animal and Plant Health Inspection Service. "Annual Report Animal Usage by Fiscal Year." June 2, 2015.
Van Zyl, Liezl. "Virtue Ethics and Right Action." In *The Cambridge Companion to Virtue Ethics*. Cambridge: Cambridge University Press, 2013.
The Vegan Option. "Lab Meat: Survey Results." May 16, 2012. http://theveganoption.org/2012/05/16/lab-meat-survey-results/.
VeganRevolution. "Brazilian Pig Eating Prank." https://www.youtube.com/watch?v=oLUAMzFqEM. Retrieved on June 26, 2014.
Vegans of Reddit. "Would Meat Grown in a Lab Change Your Mind about Eating Meat?" https://www.reddit.com/user/the_einsteinian_god. Retrieved on June 18, 2018.
Vegan Society. "We've Come a Long Way!" https://www.vegansociety.com/about-us/history. Retrieved on June 24, 2018.
"Vegetarian Dietary Patterns and Mortality in Adventist Health Study 2." *JAMA Intern. Med.* 173, no. 13 (2013): 1230–1238. doi:10.1001/jamainternmed.2013.6473.
Vegetarian Society. "Vegetarian Society Quick Polls: Lab Grown Meat. Would You Eat It?" https://www.vegsoc.org/polls.
Verbeke, Wim, Afrodita Marcu, Pieter Rutsaert, Rui Gaspar, Beate Seibt, Dave Fletcher, and Julie Barnett. "Would You Eat Cultured Meat?: Consumers' Reactions and Attitude Formation in Belgium, Portugal and the United Kingdom." *Meat Science* 102 (2015): 49–58. doi:10.1016/J.MEATSCI.2014.11.013.
Vogel, Gretchen. "Organs Made to Order." *Smithsonian.com* (August 2010). https://www.smithsonianmag.com/science-nature/organs-made-to-order-863675/. Retrieved on June 18, 2018.
Walker, Rebecca. "The Good Life for Non-Human Animals: What Virtue Requires of Humans." in *Working Virtue*, ed. Rebecca L. Walker and Philip J. Ivanhoe, 173–90. Oxford: Oxford University Press, 2007.
Warren, Mary Anne. "Difficulties With the Strong Animal Rights Position," *Between the Species* 2, no. 4 (1986). doi: https://doi.org/10.15368/bts.1986v2n4.2.
"What Is Veganism." http://animalrights.about.com/od/animalrights101/a/Veganism.htm.
White, Alex. "More Than 600,000 Animals Die Annually in Science Labs." *Herald Sun*, July 8, 2014. https://www.heraldsun.com.au/news/victoria/more-than-600000-animals-die-annually-in-science-labs/news-story/aec0d7aa495fbd7b172b2fa933399b78. Retrieved on June 12, 2018.
Why Cultured Meat – FAQ, accessed March 25, 2016; "The Crusade for a Cultured Alternative to Animal Meat: An Interview with Nicholas Genovese, PhD PETA," accessed March 25, 2016; "New Harvest – FAQ," New Harvest, accessed March 26, 2016. http://whyculturedmeat.org/faq/.
Why Cultured Meat. "Arguments." http://whyculturedmeat.org/essays/animal-rights/is-it-animal-rights/.
Williams, Bernard. *Ethics and the Limits of Philosophy*. Cambridge, MA: Harvard University Press, 1985.
———. *Utilitarianism For & Against*. Cambridge: Cambridge University Press, 1973.

Wim Verbeke, et al. "Would You Eat Cultured Meat? Consumers Reactions and Attitude Formation in Belgium, Portugal and the United Kingdom." *Meat Science* 102 (April 2015): 49–58. doi:10.1016/j.meatsci.2014.11.013.

Wood, W. Allen. "Kant on Duties Regarding Nonrational Nature." *Proceedings of the Aristotelian Society, Supplementary Volumes* 72 (1998).

Worland, Justin. "How a Vegetarian Diet Could Help Save the Planet." *Time*, March 21, 2016, http://time.com/4266874/vegetarian-diet-climate-change/. Retreived on June 14, 2018.

World Wildlife Fund. "Impact of Habitat Loss on Species." Accessed June 27, 2018. http://wwf.panda.org/our_work/wildlife/problems/habitat_loss_degradation/.

You, W., and M. Henneberg. "Meat Consumption Providing a Surplus Energy in Modern Diet Contributes to Obesity Prevalence: An Ecological Analysis" *M. BMC Nutr.* 2, no. 22 (2016). https://doi.org/10.1186/s40795-016-0063-9.

Zagzebski, Linda. *Divine Motivation Theory*. New York: Cambridge University Press, 2004.

———. "Exemplarist Virtue Theory." *Metaphilosophy* 41, no. 1/2 (2010): 41–57.

———. *Virtues of the Mind*. New York: Cambridge University Press, 1996.

———. "The Virtues of God and the Foundations of Ethics." *Faith and Philosophy* 15, no. 4 (1998): 538–553.

Index

abortion, 42, 43, 80, 111, 152, 153, 154–156, 159
absent referent, x, 118, 119
Adams, Carol J, x, 118, 139
animals, vii, viii, ix–xi, xv–xviii, xix–xxiv, 1–15, 16, 17, 18, 21, 22–23, 24, 25–26, 27, 29, 31, 35–37, 37–40, 40, 42–43, 43–44, 46–48, 49, 51, 52, 54, 55, 57, 63, 64, 75, 79–80, 81, 82, 83–85, 85, 86, 89–91, 92, 95, 96, 97, 98, 99, 99–100, 101–104, 104, 109–110, 111, 112, 113–115, 115, 116–120, 121, 125–128, 129, 130, 131–135, 136–138, 139–141, 143, 144, 146, 147, 148, 149, 150, 151, 152, 156–157, 157, 158, 159, 160, 161, 165–168, 169
Aretaic, xxi, xxii, 52, 65, 69
Aristotle, xvi, xix, 46, 55, 56, 59, 60, 62, 64, 65, 68, 71, 79, 85, 91, 92, 93, 94, 95, 97, 98, 99, 101, 104, 169

Bentham, Jeremy, 21, 22, 24, 52, 53

cancer, xi, xvii, 95, 96, 97, 121
care, vii, viii, xi, xix, xxi, xxii, xxiii, 2, 27, 31, 38, 39, 40, 42, 43, 45, 46–48, 48, 49, 52, 53, 54, 63, 69, 72, 73, 75, 79, 81, 84, 86, 90, 114, 127, 131, 134, 135, 165, 167, 168
care ethics. *See* care
carnism, 118, 137, 139, 162

Cohen, Carl, 17, 84
compassion, vii, viii, ix, xvi, xvii, xix, xxi, xxiii, 2, 28, 29, 31, 40, 43, 51, 52, 53, 54, 62, 65, 69, 70, 80, 82, 86, 91, 92, 98, 99, 100, 101, 102, 104, 109, 111, 113, 114, 115, 120, 125, 126, 127, 129, 130, 131, 132, 133, 135, 137, 138, 141, 145, 146, 161, 165, 167, 168
compassionate. *See* compassion
consequentialism, xvii, 51, 53, 54, 55, 66, 69, 71, 75, 89, 101, 129, 146
consequentialist. *See* consequentialism
cruelty, xxiii, 3, 4, 5, 7, 8, 10, 13, 52, 62, 80, 81, 90, 104, 118, 120, 129, 131, 132, 141, 146, 148, 159, 162
cultured meat, 144, 145, 147, 148, 150, 151, 152, 156, 157, 159, 160, 161

deontology, xvii, xviii, xxi, xxii, 14, 21, 23, 51, 53, 54, 55, 67, 68, 69, 89, 101, 129, 130, 145, 146, 148, 155, 165, 168
diabetes, xi, xvii–xxiii, 95, 96, 97, 121
Diamond, Cora, 36–38, 39
duty, vii, xv, xviii, xx, xxi, xxii, 1, 2, 3, 4–5, 6, 7, 8, 9, 10, 11, 12, 13, 14, 15, 16, 26, 29, 51, 52, 53, 54, 66, 67, 68, 69, 82, 83, 84, 89, 90, 101, 104, 114, 118, 130, 152, 167

empathy, viii, xxi, 29, 31, 43, 46, 52, 53, 91, 100, 130, 133, 137, 140

ethical veganism. *See* veganism
Eudaimonia, 58, 59, 62

fair. *See* fairness
fairness, vii, xxii, xxiii, 55, 92, 101, 102, 104, 109, 111, 113, 114, 132, 135, 141, 165, 167, 168
flourishing, xvi, 57, 58, 59, 62, 63, 64, 66, 70, 79, 85, 92, 109, 113, 114, 117, 121, 126, 127, 136, 138, 169
food, vii, viii, ix, x, xi, xv, xvii, xviii, xix–xx, xxiii–xxiv, 1, 11, 13, 15, 22, 23, 25, 26, 37, 38, 39, 40, 52, 55, 56, 62, 81, 83, 85, 86, 89–90, 93, 93–95, 96, 97–98, 99, 100, 101, 102, 103, 104, 109–111, 113, 114, 115, 117, 119, 120, 121, 125, 125–127, 128, 129, 131, 132, 133, 135, 137, 138, 139–140, 141, 143, 144, 146, 149, 150, 156, 157–158, 161, 162, 165–166, 168–169
Foot, Philippa, 58, 80, 81

great souled. *See* greatness of soul
greatness of soul, vii, xix, xxii, xxiii, 52, 62, 91, 92, 101, 111, 113, 127, 132, 146, 165, 167, 169

health, ix, xi, xvii–xix, xx, xxiii, 14, 26, 39, 90, 92, 93, 94, 95–96, 97, 97–98, 104, 112, 113, 117, 119, 121, 125, 137, 138, 150, 155, 156, 157, 158, 167, 169
heart disease, xi, xvii, xviii, xxiii, 95, 96, 97
Hursthouse, Rosalind, 54, 57, 60, 84, 152–154, 154, 155, 156, 159

injustice. *See* justice
intemperance. *See* temperance
Inuit, 111

Joy, Melanie, 118, 137
justice, xi, xvi, xix, xxiii, 16, 37, 45, 52, 57, 62, 71, 85, 92, 93, 99, 101, 118, 127, 130, 145, 152

Kant, Immanuel, xxii, 1, 2, 3, 4, 5, 6, 7, 8, 9, 10, 11, 12, 13, 14, 15, 21, 24, 52, 53, 58, 89, 114, 118, 167; Kantian, 2, 9, 10, 12, 13, 14, 17, 53, 69, 114, 167;

Kantianism, xxii, 18, 167; Neo-Kantian, xxii, 17, 21, 167
Kass, Leon, 159
Korsgaard Christine, xx, xxii, 9, 10, 11, 12, 13, 14, 85

lab-grown meat, 143, 144, 145, 146–147, 147, 148, 149, 150, 151, 152

Mackie, J. L., 68
magnanimity. *See* greatness of soul
marginal cases, 4, 38, 40, 42, 43, 48
McDowell, John, 58, 59
meat, viii, ix, x–xi, xvii, xix, xx, xxiii–xxiv, 26, 36, 37, 39, 52, 81, 82, 85, 90, 95, 96–97, 97, 98, 100, 102–103, 104, 109, 110–111, 115, 116, 117, 117–119, 119, 120–121, 125–126, 127, 133, 135–136, 136, 136–137, 137, 138–140, 141, 143, 144, 144–145, 146–153, 156–157, 157, 158, 159, 159–162, 165, 166
Midgley, Mary, 57, 58, 82, 95, 115, 125, 126, 159
Mill, John Stuart, xx, 21, 22, 24, 43, 44, 48
moderation, 62, 93, 95, 97, 158

nociception, 112

obesity, xi, xvii, xxii, xxiii, 97

PETA, xix, 90, 161
Preece, Gordon, 45, 82

Regan, Tom, xvii, xx, xxi, 9, 15, 16, 17, 27, 36, 80, 83, 84, 134, 135, 166
relationship, viii, xvii, xx, xxii, xxiii, xxiv, 14, 31, 37, 38, 40, 46, 47, 49, 51, 53, 64, 69, 74, 75, 82, 86, 89, 91, 92, 109, 119, 125, 126, 127, 129, 132, 133, 135, 143, 165–167

sentience. *See* sentient
sentient, xviii, 15, 21, 22, 23, 24, 25–26, 27, 31, 35, 36, 37, 41, 43, 44, 54, 86, 112, 120, 129
Singer, Peter, xvii, xx, xxi, 22, 23, 24, 25, 26, 29, 31, 35, 36, 40, 42, 43, 44, 45, 46, 47, 48, 49, 53, 54, 83, 84, 112, 134,

135, 166
subject-of-a-life, 9, 15–16, 44, 84
suffering, vii, xxi, 1, 4, 9, 12, 16, 24, 25, 26, 27, 31, 35, 36, 38, 39, 42, 44, 45, 46, 52, 54, 73, 80, 84, 85, 91, 99, 100, 102, 112, 114, 127, 129, 133, 139, 140, 143, 144, 146, 147, 148, 149, 150, 151, 152, 156, 159, 161, 162, 168

temperance, vii, viii, ix, xxii, xxiii, 52, 53, 55, 57, 62, 69, 71, 90, 92, 93, 94–95, 97–98, 101, 102, 109, 111, 114, 127, 132, 133, 138, 140, 141, 144, 145, 146, 157, 158, 161, 165, 168, 169

utilitarian. *See* utilitarianism
utilitarianism, xviii, xxii, 4, 21, 22–25, 26–30, 31, 36, 38–39, 40, 41, 43, 44, 45, 46, 48, 49, 51, 53, 53–66, 67, 68, 70, 75, 84, 101, 155, 165, 167–168

veganism, vii, viii, xv, xvi, xvii, xix, xx, xxi, xxii, xxiii, 13, 17, 52, 55, 63, 83, 84, 85, 89, 90, 91, 92, 95, 98, 99, 100, 101, 102, 104, 109, 110, 111, 112, 113, 115, 117, 119, 120, 125, 126, 127, 128, 129, 131, 133, 137, 138, 140, 143, 144, 146, 151, 161, 162, 167, 168–169
virtue, vii, viii, xi, xvi, xvii, xix, xxi, xxii, xxiii, xxiv, 3, 4, 6, 9, 17, 24, 26, 37, 44, 46, 52–54, 55–57, 59–65, 67–68, 68, 69, 69–70, 71–72, 73–75, 79–80, 81, 83–85, 86, 89–90, 91–92, 93, 97, 98, 99, 100, 100–101, 103, 104, 111, 112, 114–115, 125, 126–127, 129, 130, 131, 132, 133, 135, 137, 140, 141, 143, 145, 146, 147, 148, 152, 154, 155, 157, 159, 160, 161, 162, 165–167, 168–169
virtue ethics. *See* virtue

wisdom of repugnance, 159–160

yuck factor, 115, 116, 126, 137, 139